Care for
Hypertension

by
Neil Poulter MB BS MSc FRCP
Professor of Preventive Cardiovascular Medicine, Cardiovascular Studies Unit, Imperial College School of Medicine at St Mary's, London, UK

Simon Thom MB BS MD FRCP
Reader, Department of Clinical Pharmacology, Imperial College School of Medicine at St Mary's, London, UK

Michael Kirby MB BS LRCP MRCS FRCP
Family Practitioner, The Surgery, Letchworth, UK and Director, HertNet (The Hertfordshire Primary Care Research Network), Hertfordshire, UK

ISIS
MEDICAL
MEDIA

A division of Health Media Limited
Finsbury Tower
103–105 Bunhill Row
London EC1Y 8LZ

First published 2001

British Library Cataloguing-in-Publication Data.
A catalogue record for this title is available from the British Library.

ISBN 1 899066 80 2

Poulter, N, Thom, S, Kirby, M
Shared Care for Hypertension

Always refer to the manufacturer's Prescribing Information before prescribing drugs cited in this book.

Indexing
Laurence Errington

Medical art
Oxford Illustrators

Design, illustrations and typesetting
InPerspective Ltd.

Isis Medical Media staff
Publisher: John Harrison
Senior Editorial Controller: Sarah Carlson
Production & Editorial Manager: Julia Savory
Production Manager: Sarah Sodhi

Produced by Phoenix Offset, HK
Printed in China

Distributed in the USA by
Books International, Inc., P.O. Box 605,
Herndon, VA 20172, USA

Distributed in the rest of the world by
Plymbridge Distributors Ltd., Estover Road,
Plymouth PL6 7PY, UK

Contents

Preface

Globally, hypertension is one of the most common preventable risk factors accounting for ill health and mortality. The risk of coronary heart disease and stroke is directly related to elevated blood pressure levels, and these cardiovascular diseases will become the world's commonest cause of premature death within the next decade

We know that, in practice, the detection of hypertension is inadequate, thresholds for intervention in high-risk patients are inappropriately high and achievement of target blood pressures in those that are treated is the exception rather than the rule. Recent surveys suggest that the situation is improving – at least in Western countries - but current guidelines are moving the goal posts to yet lower threshold and target levels. Hence there remains room for improvement.

The chronic nature of hypertension and the diversity of associated complications mean that the medical care of any patient with this condition is a long-term process involving several different professional skills. This book aims to define the integration of general and specialist aspects of hypertension management.

The book is intended as a guide for all health-care professionals involved in the care of people with hypertension. The text covers the epidemiology of hypertension, diagnosis, investigation and the expanding range of pharmacological and non-pharmacological treatments. Although the NHS in the UK provides a natural focus for the authors, the basic principles of shared care are applicable worldwide. This is essentially a practical guide to shared hypertension care references are kept to a minimum but ideas for further reading are included. We hope it will be useful to the many physicians and nurses in primary and secondary care who face the daily challenge of diagnosing and managing this most prevalent disorder.

Neil Poulter
Simon Thom
Mike Kirby
January 2001

Abbreviations

ABPM	ambulatory blood pressure monitoring
ACE	angiotensin-converting enzyme
AII	angiotensin II
BHS	British Hypertension Society
BMI	body mass index
BP	blood pressure
BPH	benign prostatic hypertrophy
CAPPP	Captopril Prevention Project
CCF	congestive cardiac failure
CHD	coronary heart disease
COPD	chronic obstructive pulmonary disease
CT	computed tomography
CV	cardiovascular
CVA	cerebrovascular accident
CVD	cardiovascular disease
CVS	cardiovascular system
DM	diabetes mellitus
ECG	electrocardiograph/electrocardiography
Echo	echocardiograph
ED	erectile disfunction
FVR	forearm vascular resistance
γGTP	gamma glutamyl transpeptidase
HDL	high-density lipoprotein
HRT	hormone replacement therapy
IGT	impaired glucose intolerance
ISH	isolated systolic hypertension
JNC VI	Joint National Committee VI
LDL	low-density lipoprotein
LV	left ventricular
LVH	left ventricular hypertrophy
MCV	mean corpuscular volume
MRI	magnetic resonance imaging
NSF	National Service Framework
OC	oral contraceptive
PAI-1	platelet activator inhibitor 1
PHCT	primary health-care team
PPARγ	peroxisome proliferator activator receptor
PVD	peripheral vascular disease
SYST-EUR	Systolic Hypertension – Europe Trial
UKPDS	United Kingdom Prospective Diabetes Study
WHO–ISH	World Health Organization – International Society of Hypertension

chapter 1

Size of the problem

INTRODUCTION

Hypertension remains a major health-care concern in western industrialized countries. Indeed, in the USA alone, nearly 50 million people have elevated blood pressure (BP) that warrants some form of treatment or monitoring. In this chapter a concise overview of the scale of the problem is presented. The significant morbidity and mortality that arise from the cardiovascular sequelae of hypertension, such as stroke and myocardial infarction, are discussed elsewhere in this book (see Chapter 5).

BP levels are normally distrubuted in the population (Fig. 1.1). It is also clear that no distinct subset of the population appear to be abnormal from a BP viewpoint, and that the prevalence of hypertension is highly dependent upon the level of BP at which hypertension is defined (Fig. 1.1).

In 1968 Pickering said hypertension is 'a disorder hitherto unrecognized in medicine, in which the defect is qualitative and not quantitative. It is difficult for doctors to understand because it is a departure from the ordinary process of binary thought to which they are brought up. Medicine in its present state can count up to two, but not beyond.'

Not much has changed in 32 years, in that there is still a tendency to consider hypertension as present or absent, and this clearly has major implications for exactly how hypertension is defined.

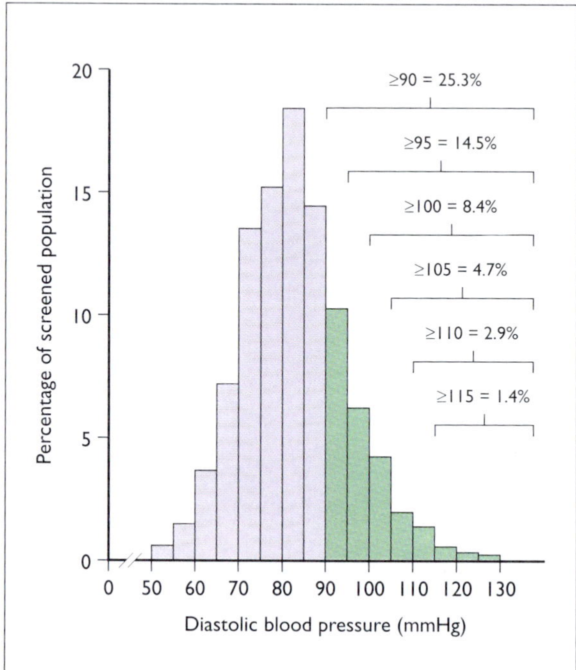

Figure 1.1. Distribution of BP in the population.

DEFINITION OF HYPERTENSION

There are several ways to classify and define the levels of BP that might be considered as 'hypertensive', of which one possible set is summarized in Table 1.1. However, the decision processes whereby these definitions are determined are, to an extent, unscientific and arbitrary. Risk of adverse cardiovascular sequelae such as stroke or acute myocardial infarction shows a continuous linear relationship with increasing levels of diastolic (Fig. 1.2) or systolic BP. Consequently, from a prognostic viewpoint no obvious level of BP clearly separates normal ('normotension') from abnormal ('hypertension'). One classic method of defining abnormal levels of a biological variable is to use the level beyond two standard deviations above the mean. The weakness of this method is that all populations would have a prevalence of hypertension of 5%, irrespective of the actual levels of BP. The pragmatic approach to defining hypertension derives

Table 1.1. Definitions and classification of BP levels. WHO–ISH (1999) in line with JNC VI [3, 4]

Category	Systolic (mmHg)	Diastolic (mmHg)
Optimal	<120	<80
Normal	<130	<85
High–normal	130–139	85–89
Hypertension		
Grade 1 (mild)	140–159	90–99
Subgroup borderline	140–149	90–94
Grade 2 (moderate)	160–179	100–109
Grade 3 (severe)	≥180	≥110
Isolated systolic hypertension	≥140	<90
Subgroup borderline	140–149	<90

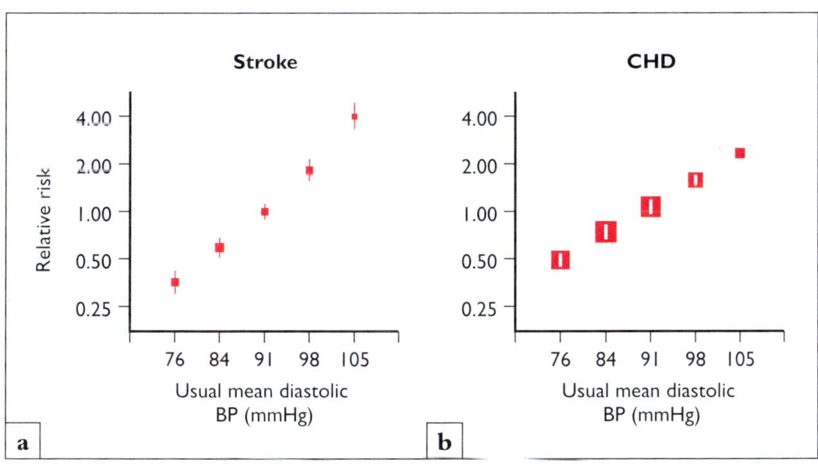

Figure 1.2. Risk of (a) stroke (seven prospective observational studies, 843 events) or (b) coronary heart disease (CHD) (nine prospective observational studies, 4856 events) with level of diastolic BP.

mainly from trial evidence that clearly establishes the benefits, in terms of reduced cardiovascular events, of lowering BP (see Chapter 12). Hence a working definition becomes:

Hypertension is that level of BP above which investigation and treatment do more good than harm.

In recent years several sets of national and international guidelines on the detection, evaluation and management of hypertension have been produced [1–5] and they have all proposed thresholds of systolic and/or diastolic BP above which therapy should be initiated once sufficient BP measurements had been made.

The guidelines are reasonably consistent in that they all recommend drug intervention at systolic BP ≥160 mmHg or ≥100 mmHg diastolic BP in those patients with no other major risk factors. These sets of guidelines recognize, as do the definitions shown in Table 1.1, that systolic BP levels should receive at least the same attention as diastolic BP levels when considering hypertension treatment. Historically, diastolic BP has been the focus of attention and the importance of systolic BP has been underrated. It is now reasonably clear that systolic is probably a better predictor of cardiovascular disease than diastolic BP and hence the contemporary recommendation that both systolic and diastolic BP should be considered, and that elevation of either merits intervention.

One legacy from the past, which should be discarded, is that normal and acceptable systolic BP can be calculated by adding the age in years to 100. This obviously assumes that it is normal for BP to rise with age. It is true that it is usual for BP to rise with age (Fig. 1.3), but only in populations in which it is usual (or common) to die of CHD or stroke. The 'normal' rise of BP with age is the result of pathological changes in the vasculature and the truly normal situation – as observed in countries in which CHD and stroke are non-endemic – is one in which BP does not rise with age (Fig. 1.4). In these 'low-BP populations' hypertension

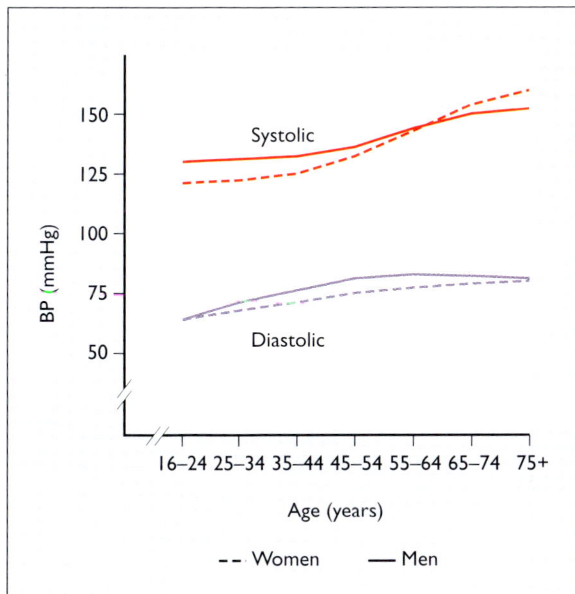

Figure 1.3. Mean BP levels amongst English adults by age (data from [8]).

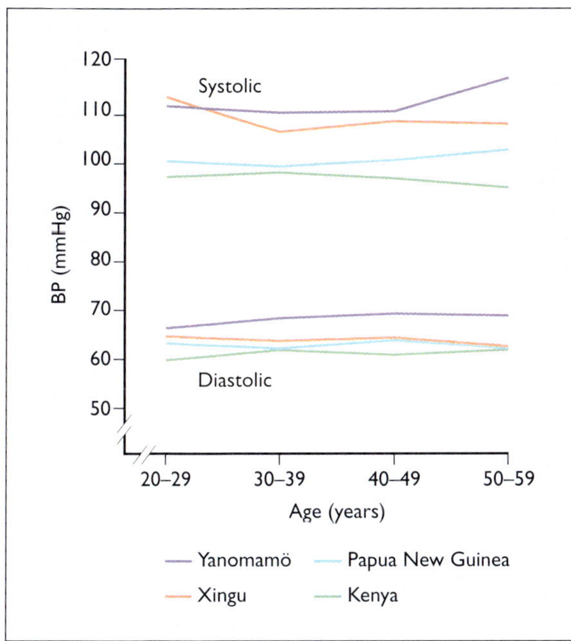

Figure 1.4. Line graphs of systolic and diastolic pressures by 10-year age groups in four low BP populations [15].

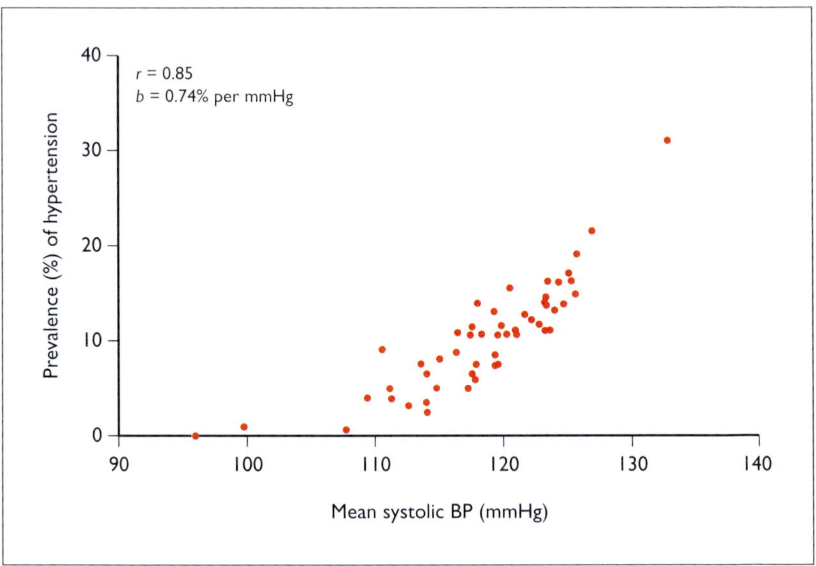

Figure 1.5. Relationship between population mean systolic BP and the prevalence of hypertension across 52 population samples from 32 countries [10].

is either extremely rare or non-existent, consistent with the observation that the rate of rise of BP with age in a population correlates with the prevalence of hypertension, as does the mean BP level of a population (Fig. 1.5).

Prevalence of hypertension

The prevalence of hypertension varies dramatically among different populations around the world. In some populations, essential hypertension is completely absent [6] whereas in others, such as some black populations in the USA, the majority of adults are considered hypertensive [7].

In the UK, recent large national surveys in England and Scotland [8, 9] – the *Health Survey for England*, and the *Scottish Health Survey* – included evaluations of BP levels among a representative sample of the adult populations. The prevalence of hypertension in England and Scotland (defined as a systolic BP ≥160 mmHg, a diastolic BP ≥95 mmHg or being on treatment for hypertension), as evaluated in these two surveys, was about 18% in England (age ≥16 years) [11] and 11.9% in Scotland (age 16–64 years).

Thus, almost one-fifth of adults over 16 years of age in the UK are 'hypertensive'. BP tends to be higher among men than women up to the age of about 55 years, after which women have higher pressures. Also, BP shows a geographical gradient, being higher in the north than in the south [8], and tend to be higher in lower socioeconomic strata, particularly among women. However, the differences in BP that are associated with socioeconomic factors appear to be explained largely by higher levels of body mass index in men and women from lower social strata and, among men, by the higher alcohol intakes of those in lower social strata [12]. Finally, BP levels are higher in ethnic minority groups, particularly the African–Caribbean population and, to a lesser extent, the South Asian population [13].

These high levels of hypertension in the UK population clearly constitute a huge problem in terms of the associated disease burden and the costs of health care. It is therefore totally appropriate that a target to lower average systolic BP by the year 2005 was set in the Government's 1992 strategy document, the *Health of the Nation* [14]. It was reassuring that mean BP levels in England moved in the right direction until 1994, but thereafter this trend has stopped, and if current trends in BP continue, the *Health of the Nation* targets will not be met.

As Figure 1.3 implies, the prevalence of isolated systolic hypertension tends to be higher in older age groups. Furthermore, given the ever-increasing longevity of the UK population, isolated systolic hypertension is increasingly encountered in clinical practice (see Chapter 10).

Chapter Summary

- The prevalence of hypertension is highly dependent on the level of BP at which hypertension is defined.
- A working definition becomes: 'hypertension is that level of BP above which investigation and treatment do more good than harm'.
- Almost one-fifth of the adult population in the UK are hypertensive (≥160mmHg SBP or ≥ 95mmHg DBP).
- Hypertension is a large public health problem throughout the world.
- There is a strong causal relationship between hypertension and cardiovascular disease.
- Recent national and international guidelines are reasonably consistent and recognize that systolic BP levels should receive at least the same attention as diastolic BP levels.
- The 'normal rise' of BP with age is the result of pathological changes in the vasculature.
- With demographic changes in the population, isolated systolic hypertension is increasingly encountered in clinical practice.
- Prevention of stroke and coronary heart disease are key targets in the *Health of the Nation, Our Healthier Nation* and the *National Service Framework* publications.

References

1. Myers MG, Carruthers SG, Leenen FHH, Haynes RB. Recommendations from the Canadian Hypertension Society Consensus Conference on the pharmacologic treatment of hypertension. *Can Med Assoc J* 1989; **140**: 1141–6.
2. Jackson R, Barham P, Bills J, *et al*. Management of raised blood pressure in New Zealand: a discussion document. *BMJ* 1993; **307**: 107–10.

3. 1999 World Health Organization – International Society of Hypertension guidelines for the management of hypertension. *Blood Pressure* 1999; **8**: 1–43.
4. Joint National Committee on Detection, Evaluation and Treatment of High Blood Pressure. The sixth report of the Joint National Committee on Prevention, Detection, Evaluation and Treatment of High Blood Pressure (JNCVI). *Arch Intern Med* 1997; **157**: 2413–46.
5. Ramsay LE, Johnston GD, MacGregor GA, *et al.* Guidelines for management of hypertension: report of the third working party of the British Hypertension Society. *J Hum Hypertens* 1999; **13**: 569–92.
6. Poulter NR, Sever PS. Low blood pressure populations and the impact of rural urban migration. In: Swales J, ed. *Textbook of Hypertension*. Oxford: Blackwell Scientific Publications Ltd, 1994.
7. Kaplan NM, Venkata C, Ram S. Hypertension in ethnic subgroups. In: Swales J, ed. *Textbook of Hypertension*. Oxford: Blackwell Scientific Publications Ltd, 1994.
8. Colhoun H, Prescott-Clarke P, eds, and Joint Health Surveys Team on behalf of the Department of Health. *Health Survey for England 1994*, Vols I and II. London: HMSO, 1996.
9. Dong W, Erens B, eds, and Joint Health Surveys Unit on behalf of the Department of Health. *Scottish Health Survey 1995*. Edinburgh: The Stationery Office, 1997.
10. Rose G. *The Strategy of Preventive Medicine*. Oxford: Oxford University Press, 1992.
11. Colhoun HM, Dong W, Poulter NR. Blood pressure screening, management and control in England: results from the Health Survey for England 1994. *J Hypertens* 1998; **16**: 747–53.
12. Colhoun HM, Hemingway H, Poulter NR. Socioeconomic status and blood pressure: a systematic overview. *J Hum Hypertens* 1998; **12**: 91–110.
13. Primatesta P, Bost L, Poulter NR. Blood pressure levels and hypertension status among ethnic groups in England. *J Hum Hypertens* 2000; **14**: 143–8.
14. Department of Health. *The Health of the Nation: a strategy for health in England*. London: HMSO, 1992.
15. Carvalho JJ, Baruzzi RG, Howard PF, *et al.* Blood pressure in four remote populations in the INTERSALT Study. *Hypertension* 1989; **14**: 238–46.

chapter 2

Concepts, implications and applications of shared care

The management of the hypertensive patient is an undertaking that is likely to involve a considerable amount of two- and three-way dialogue between patient and their physicians (a generalist and a specialist; Fig. 2.1). Potentially, unless the process of patient management is carried out effectively and efficiently from day one, the potential for a high degree of duplication of effort by general practitioner and specialist is considerable [1]. In an attempt to rationalize patient management and minimize unnecessary resource waste and duplication, shared care is being increasingly employed in the UK and Europe. The long-term management of patients with hypertension does, and will increasingly, present substantial problems for health-care providers with respect to numbers [2] and the poor rate of compliance and/or high rate of drop-out during follow-up [3]. A shared care approach may provide some solutions.

Six key components must be fulfilled for any shared care scheme in any country to be successful:

- Government endorsement and support
- A viable national health-care infrastructure
- Available local facilities and resources

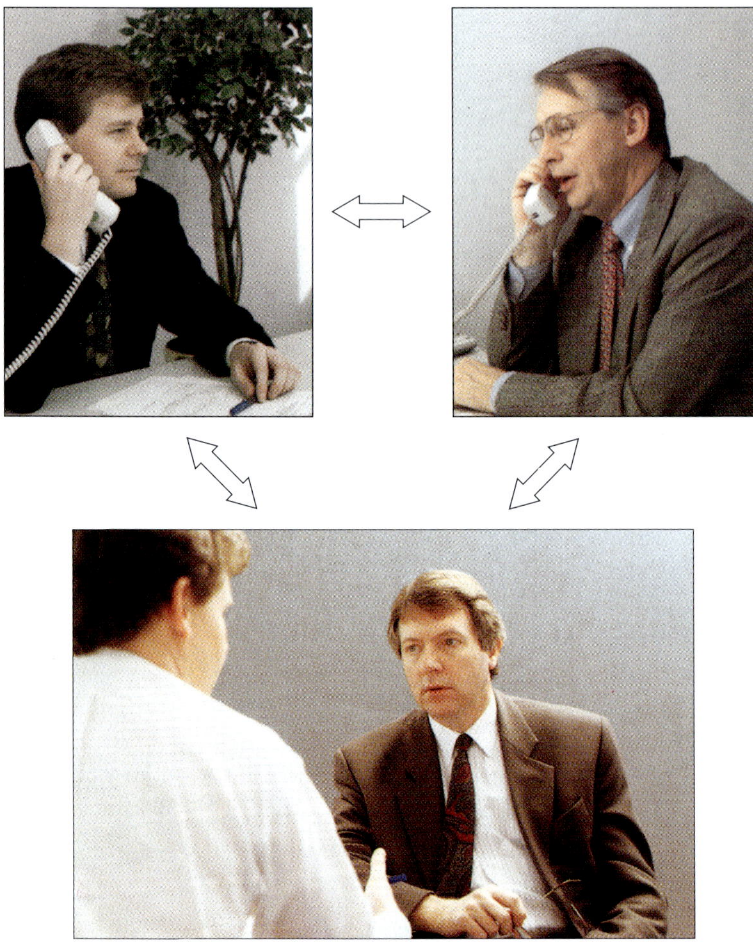

Figure 2.1. Three-way communication.

- Community practitioners with shared care experience
- Established viable working relationship between community practitioners and specialists
- Availability of other community-based health-care professionals.

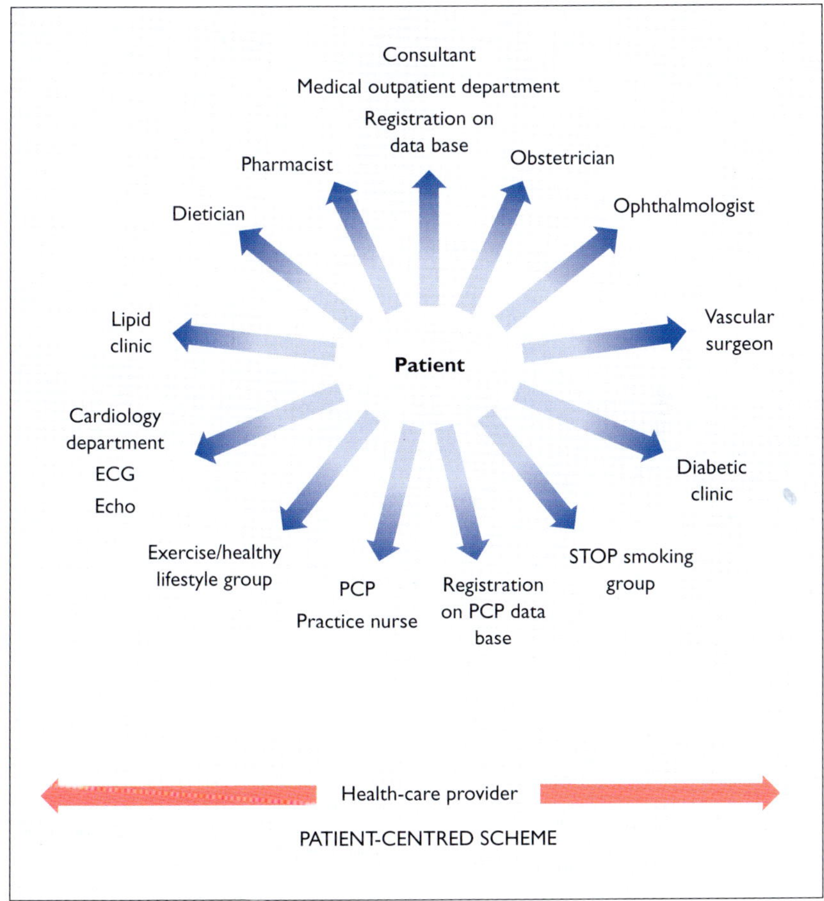

Figure 2.2. Anatomy of a shared care scheme. PCP; primary care practice.

Shared care (Fig 2.2) [4] has been defined as:

> *The joint participation of hospital consultants and general practitioners in the planned delivery of care for patients with a chronic condition, informed by an enhanced information exchange over and above routine discharge and referral notices.*

In view of the demographics of hypertension, discussed in Chapter 1, and the staffing pressures within the hospital systems in many countries, the implication of shared care is attractive and should be well received. With an increase in detection rate, because of population screening policies, and the increasing percentage of elderly subjects in many populations, the sheer number of new cases alone could swamp most countries' health-care systems. Apart from the potential impact on health-care resource utilization, shared care should also improve the continuity of care for the elderly and post-stroke patients who may find it difficult to attend hospital clinics.

The advantages of shared care to patients, primary care physicians, specialists and health-care providers are listed below.

Advantages for patients

- A reduction in the number of hospital visits and shorter referral time
- Easier access to medical advice at all levels
- Greater continuity of treatment
- More contact with the family doctor, who has a more complete knowledge of the medical and social issues for each patient.

Advantages for primary care physicians

- Reduction in the consequences of untreated hypertension within the practice
- Patients may be more open with a familiar health-care professional (family doctor or practice nurse)
- Opportunity to broaden knowledge and develop new skills in a particular area of medicine and disease management
- Team work is often more rewarding.

Advantages for specialists

- Reduction in hospital admissions
- More appropriate specialist referral
- More time available for patients who require specialist management
- Improved relations between primary care physicians and specialists.

Advantages for health-care providers

- Integrated approach provides more efficient use of finite resources
- Provides continuity of treatment and ensures patient well-being in the long term
- Team building for future initiatives
- Consistent with Government policies
- Provides a basis for evaluation and audit.

SHARED-CARE PROGRAMMES

There is now an added incentive to the instigation of shared-care programmes, in that several countries have espoused or will shortly espouse policies that include devolution of chronic disease management from secondary to primary care physicians [5, 6]. In countries such as the USA the major health-care providers (insurance companies) have already implemented such a move on the basis of economics.

The function and viability of any multidisciplinary team depends on setting well-defined objectives .The roles of the participants must be defined precisely and unequivocally; the participants must also feel empowered and yet accountable, and should trust one another implicitly. In view of the considerable level of delineation and demarcation involved, cross-divisional communication and collaboration is the key to ensuring an efficient, integrated approach.The prime clinical objective is well controlled blood pressure in a greater number of hypertensive patients.

Shared care has been implemented successfully in the USA and in several European countries.The UK has been in the vanguard of implementing this new approach [7–9]. Here, initiative in coordinating the care of hypertensive patients attending hospitals and the provision of advice on appropriate treatments and follow-up regimes has been driven by hospital departments.The original objectives in the 1980s were to improve communication between hospitals and general practices, to share experiences and expertise and to reduce the frequency of hospital visits. These objectives have been met with a considerable degree of success in the centres involved.

In other countries, particularly the USA, as a result of a different infrastructure, the large health-care providers undertake the integration of all activities. The philosophy of shared care in general practice, based partly on the success of the hypertension model, has become widely accepted and is being extended into the long-term management of other diseases. It is therefore logical that the coordination of shared care for hypertension should evolve to a system driven by the primary care physicians rather than the hospital.

Increasing numbers of primary care physicians now have computers to enable the registration of patient details and health status. In addition, automated appointment setting, clinical algorithms and medication details are available, and there are major opportunities for data acquisition and transfer via internet access and e-mail. Such facilities provide the structure to comply with any national or international guidelines [9]. One example is PRODIGY, which offers primary care physicians practical support by providing authoritative, relevant clinical and prescribing advice through their desktop computer. e-MIMMS has also recently become widely available – in the UK up to 38% of primary care physicians were using the system according to a market research survey in July 1999.

Doctors use such systems during consultations and are offered guidance tailored to individual patients using information from the electronic patient record. As well as therapeutic recommendations, guidance may include patient information leaflets and advice on referral or investigation. Such systems also include supporting information, for example, references and the rationale behind treatment selection, that can be accessed outside of consultation for educational purposes [10]. A number of tools are available to enhance the doctor–patient relationship: as well as patient information leaflets, there are screens that contain advice for primary physicians to share with patients during consultations. The aim of these automated systems is to support the primary physician, who is able to adapt the clinical recommendations to reflect local treatment preferences.

Successful implementation of guidelines often depends heavily on local ownership and the local adaptation of national guidelines to accommodate practice protocol guidelines. The devolution of some additional responsibility to practice nurses and other members of the primary health-care team (PHCT) facilitates implementation. Within the protocol there must be, as a minimum, clear definition as to when the patient is referred to the general practitioner, who may decide on appropriate further investigation or to change treatment plans or when consultant referral is required. In the UK the majority of hypertensive patients are managed in the primary care setting, with <10% referral to a specialist. Specialist advice may be required in the situations described below [11].

SUGGESTED INDICATIONS FOR SPECIALIST REFERRAL [11]

Urgent treatment needed

- Accelerated (malignant) hypertension
- More severe hypertension (e.g. >220/120 mmHg)
- Complications (e.g. transient ischaemic attack, left ventricular failure).

Possible underlying cause

- Any clue in history or examination of a secondary cause:
- Hypokalaemia and increased plasma sodium (Conn's syndrome?)
- Elevated serum creatinine
- Proteinuria or haematuria
- Recent onset or worsening of hypertension
- Resistant to a three-drug regimen
- Young age (any hypertension in patient <20 years old; any patient who needs treatment and is <30 years old).

Therapeutic problems

- Treatment resistance
- Multiple drug intolerance
- Multiple drug contraindications
- Persistent noncompliance
- Treatment declined (the reluctant hypertensive).

Special situations

- Unusual BP variability
- Possible 'white-coat' hypertension
- Hypertension in pregnancy.

After resolution by the consultant

Subsequent to problem resolution by the consultant, the patient then returns to the primary care setting for further follow-up.

The operations of some of the smaller health-care providers in the USA with regard to the management of hypertension are well worth careful scrutiny by those considering setting up a shared-care programme.

Devolution of responsibility

The keys to success of a shared-care programme are:

- Integrated training for specialist and the PHCT
- Development of a formal local protocol of patient management (see Tables 8.15 and 7.9)
- Good communications between all members of the team involved in patient care
- Easy, guaranteed access to the specialist's advice
- Motivation of the specialist towards community involvement
- Ease of use by patients
- Practice nurses familiar with management of hypertension
- Ownership of the scheme by all participants.

Although shared care results in a shift in responsibility for disease management from hospitals to general practices, this is not the most important shift in emphasis. As exemplified by the experience in asthma and diabetes, practice nurses are the key to successful patient management. In essence they become the practice experts in the management of some chronic conditions and the front line in the interface between patients and the local medical system. As such, practice nurses must be fully empowered to carry out this major task to the best of their ability.

A key component of any shared-care system is to hold educational meetings within the health-care provider community. These meetings are essential to share ideas, to solve problems in groups and to promote education and research. Obviously, underpinning the whole operation are knowledge about local guidelines for patient management and a good understanding of logistics and tactics of implementation. Outside the group, responsibility has to be taken for patient education and increasing disease awareness using national, local and contemporary material. In particular, background material on the importance of cardiovascular risk factors and options of treatment (lifestyle modification and pharmacological intervention) should be made available to patients and partners. Systems used to generate letters from hypertension clinics and primary-care computer systems could be used to provide a unified structure of information and advice, and to speed up the dissemination of additional information to patients.

Assuming that the hypertensive patient presents and participates in a disease-management programme, this need not be their only level of involvement. Patient-held cards enable the patients to feel part of the team by making them feel additionally accountable for their progress towards personal health targets, which will undoubtedly include lifestyle modification. Thus, the patient is a key player in the management team. Compliance is one of the most important factors affecting the success of hypertension management – a retrospective analysis of hypertensive patients being treated in general practice found that 50–59% of patients discontinued their treatment after only 6 months of therapy [12]. Poor compliance may in part account for the high percentage of hypertensive patients who are, in theory, being treated and yet who remain uncontrolled. It is important to identify such patients and reviewing the frequency of the collection of repeat prescriptions is an ideal way to address this problem.

How to improve compliance:

- Ensure the patient understands the reasons and benefits of treatment
- Give clear instructions
- Repeat and reinforce instructions at each visit
- Inquire about side effects
- Put treatment regimes and objectives in writing
- Keep the treatment simple
- Prefer once-day dosing where possible
- Avoid mid-day dosing where possible
- Reinforce patient's participation in his/her own care
- Involve the patient's relatives, especially for the elderly patient
- Involve the practice nurse in regular follow-up.

Conclusion

The benefits of a shared care approach to the management of hypertension to patients, general physicians, specialists and shared care providers are well known. In the UK, elsewhere in Europe and in the USA, shared care schemes have been successfully implemented and have had major impacts on both health-care costs and on patient's quality of life. Given this experience, the shared-care approach to the management of hypertension can be adopted with confidence.

Chapter Summary

- Shared care is 'the joint participation of hospital consultants and the PHCT in the planned delivery of care of patients with hypertension'; it involves enhanced information exchange over and above the usual referral and discharge letters.
- Health promotion now has a firm footing in primary care.
- There are advantages for the patient, primary care physician, specialist and health-care providers in undertaking a shared care approach.
- Shared care is applicable to the other diseases that may be concomitant.
- Computerization facilitates shared care and can be used to provide a unified structure, particularly when decision support systems and guidelines are incorporated.
- Local ownership is critical to the success.
- Practice nurses are the key to a successful outcome.
- Educational meetings within the PHCT and in the locality are important.
- Patient health cards can be helpful.
- A written protocol is needed for the PHCT.
- Educational support must be given for the PHCT.
- Compliance with treatment and medical advice is one of the most important factors to determine the success or failure of BP control.
- In the UK, the advent of primary care groups and trusts provide an ideal opportunity to set up a shared-care scheme for hypertension.
- Shared care is being increasingly employed in the USA, UK and Europe.

References

1. Parkins DM, Kellet RJ, MacLean DW, *et al.* The management of hypertension – a study of records in general practice. *J Coll Gen Pract* 1979; **29**: 590–4.
2. 1999 World Health Organization – International Society of Hypertension guidelines for the management of hypertension. Guidelines subcommittee. *J Hypertens* 1999; **17**: 151–83.
3. Bullpit CJ, Raymond MJ, Dollery CT. Community care compared with hospital out-patient care for hypertensive patients. *BMJ* 1982; **284**: 554–6.
4. Hickman M, Drummond N, Grimshaw J. A taxonomy of shared care for chronic disease. *J Public Health Med* 1994; **16**: 447–54.
5. Hughes J, Gordon P. *Hospitals and Primary Care – Breaking the Boundaries.* London: Kings Fund Centre, 1992.
6. Glucklick C. *The Extent of the Movement of Acute Services from the Hospital to the Primary and Community Care.* London: Kings Fund Centre, 1994.
7. McGhee SM, McInnes GT, Hedley AJ *et al.* Coordinating and standardizing long-term care: evaluation of the west of Scotland shared-care scheme for hypertension. *Br J Gen Pract* 1994; **44**: 441–5.
8. Petrie JC, Robb OJ, Webster J, *et al.* Computer assisted shared care in hypertension. *Br Med J* 1985; **290**:1960–62.
9. Petrie JC, Webster J, Jeffers TA, *et al.* Computer assisted shared care. *J Hypertens* 1989; **7(Suppl 3)**: S103–8.
10. Purves IN. PRODIGY: implementing clinical guidance using computers. *Br J Gen Pract* 1998; 48: 1552–3.
11. Ramsay LE, Johnston GD, MacGregor GA, *et al.* Guidelines for management of hypertension: report of the third working party of the British Hypertension Society. *J Hum Hypertens* 1999; **13**: 569–92.
12. Jones JK, Gorkin L, Lian JF, *et al.* Discontinuation of, and changes in, treatment after start of new courses of anti-hypertensive drugs: a study of a United Kingdom population. *BMJ* 1995; **311**: 293–5.

chapter 3

Blood pressure measurement

INTRODUCTION

Accurate and reliable measurements of BP are essential for the diagnosis of hypertension and monitoring the response to therapy. Measurements of BP were first made and recorded more than 250 years ago. In this chapter a concise overview of the history and practice of BP measurement is presented.

The site at which BP is measured has a significant effect on the observed reading. Figure 3.1 presents a simplified illustration of the regulation of BP within the cardiovascular system, while Figure 3.2 shows the sequential changes in pressure that occur along the branches of the vascular tree. The brachial artery is most commonly used as the site of measurement. The range of values considered to be normal are between 90 and 129 mmHg for systolic BP and between 60 and 84 mmHg for diastolic BP.

MEASUREMENT METHODS

Techniques for the measurement of BP have a long and fascinating history. The Anglican cleric Stephen Hales was the first to describe direct BP measurement in both the systemic and pulmonary circulations of several species. He inserted a brass cannula in the carotid artery of a horse and connected this via a flexible tube to a glass manometer. Using this apparatus he demonstrated that blood rose to a height

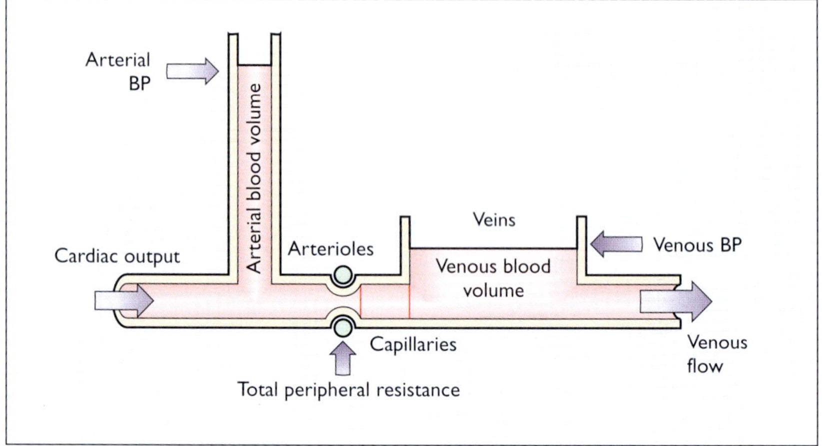

Figure 3.1. The regulation of BP within the cardiovascular system.

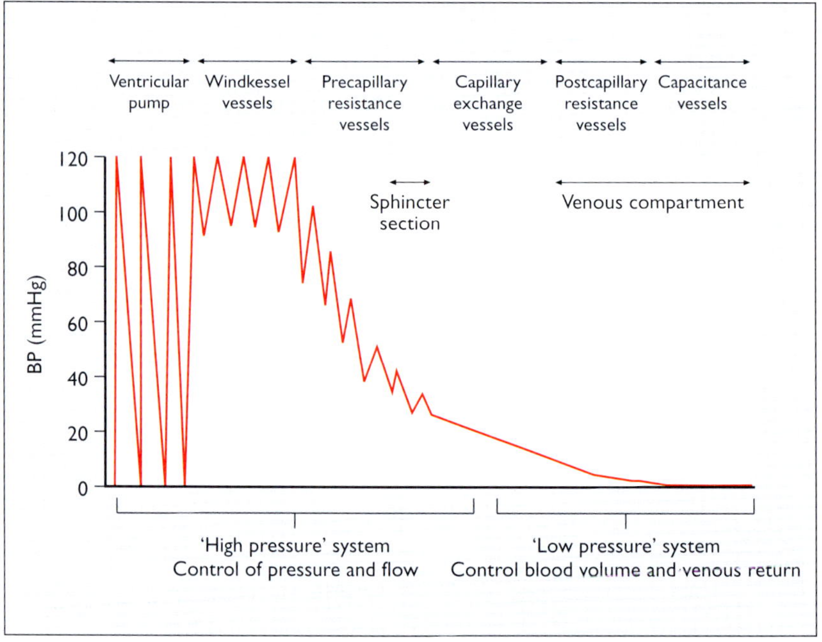

Figure 3.2. Sequential changes in BP occurring along branches of the vascular tree.

of 9 feet above the heart (Fig. 3.3). Since the relative densities of blood and mercury (Hg) are about 1.06 and 13.6 respectively, Hales' figures are equivalent to a pressure of 225 mmHg. This is much higher than

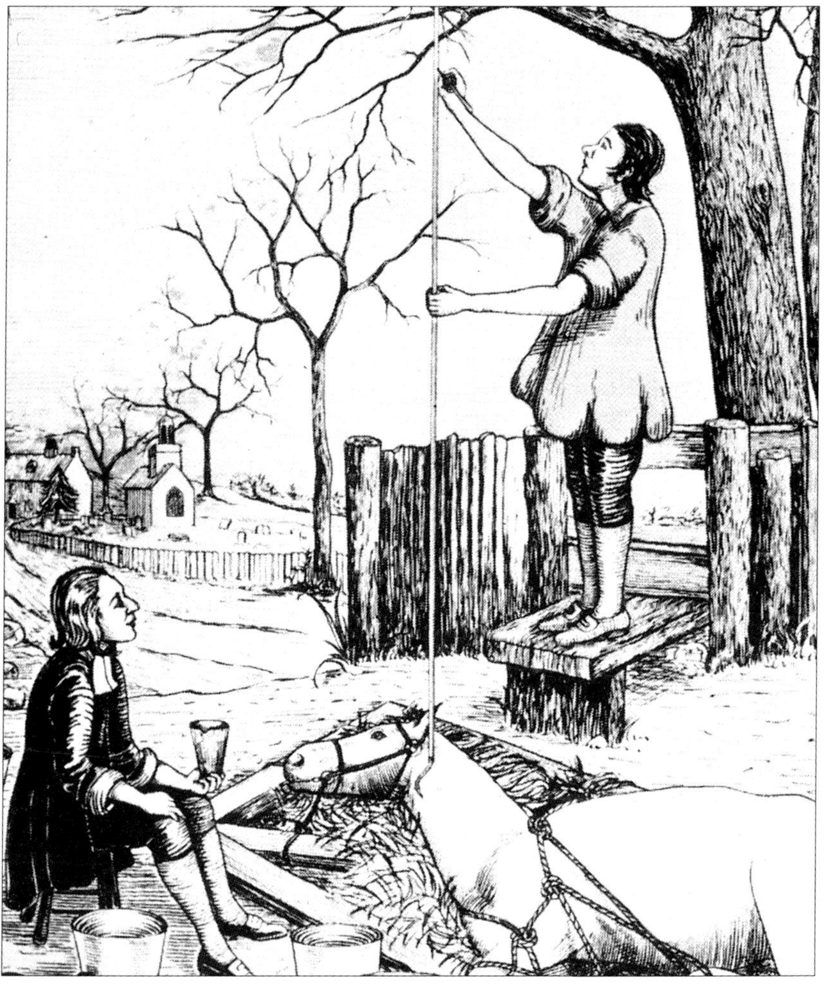

Figure 3.3. Hales making manometric measurements from the carotid artery of a horse in 1733.

the normal equine BP of 120 mmHg and may reflect the fact that Hales' horse was unanaesthetized!

More than a century later Frederick Mahomed modified a prototype 'sphygmograph' which allowed readings of systolic BP. Marey recorded the pulse wave by applying a tambour and lever system over the artery and used a plunger just proximal to the tambour to apply measured amounts of pressure. The method was greatly simplified by Riva-Rocci in 1896 by using a cuff placed round the arm. Scipione Riva-Rocci devised the air-filled rubber bladder as an occlusive cuff for the measurement of systolic pressure.

In 1905 Nicolai Korotkoff observed the bruits generated in the brachial artery below the Riva-Rocci cuff that provide the basis for an accurate determination of both systolic and diastolic pressures. The principle is to determine the pressure that must be applied to the artery to make the pulse disappear at a point distal to the application of pressure. This idea developed from a practice of nineteenth-century physicians, who used three fingers to assess the quality of the pulse in palpable arteries. The flow was occluded by the most distal, the pulse was felt by the middle finger and the pressure exerted by the finger proximal to the heart was varied. A pump inflated the cuff until it acted like a tourniquet to cut off blood flow. A mercury manometer measured the pressure in the cuff. The pressure was then gently lowered and it was noted when the pulse reappeared in the brachial or radial artery below the cuff. The device is called a sphygmomanometer from the Greek *sphygmos,* meaning pulse. The Korotkoff modification involved the description of sounds heard in the stethoscope applied over the palpable artery (Fig. 3.4). As the pressure in the cuff is lowered the first sounds, which correspond to the reappearance of the pulse, are produced by spurts of blood impinging on the stationary column of blood below the point of occlusion. The first sounds occur when the peaks of systolic pressure just exceed the pressure used to occlude the artery. As the pressure of the cuff is lowered, the sounds become muffled and disappear altogether when the occlusion pressure equals the diastolic pressure (Fig. 3.5). This auscultatory method aided by a mercury manometer survives to this day.

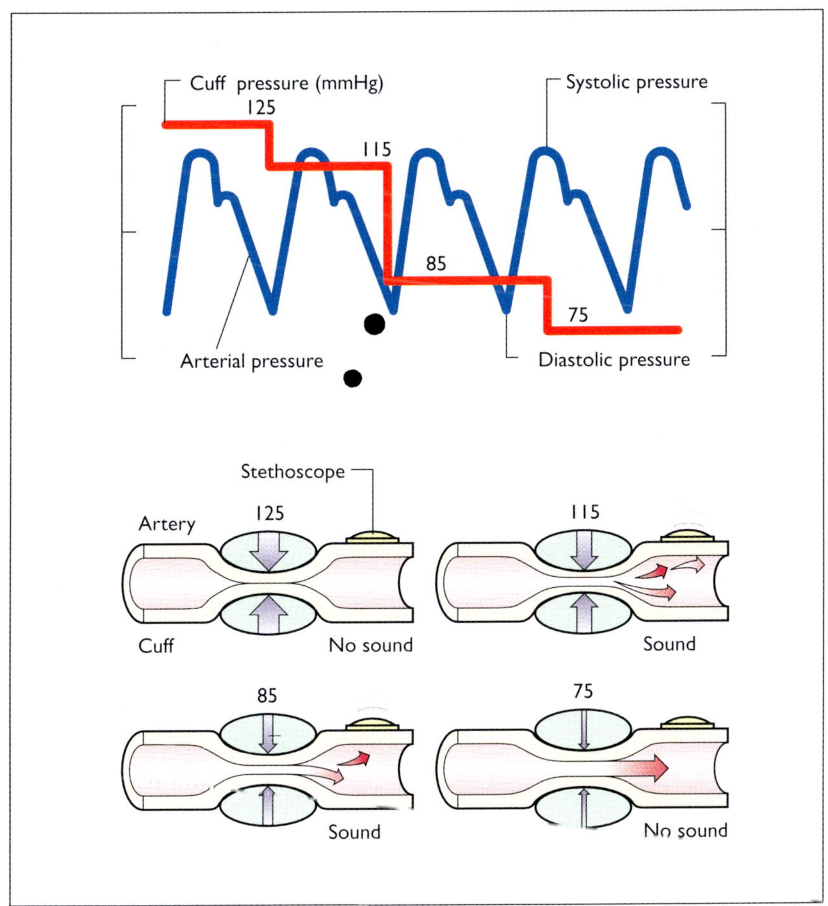

Figure 3.4. Sounds heard with application of the stethoscope over the palpable artery.

The forthcoming environmental safety policy within Europe to remove mercury from general use means that we face imminent changes in BP measurement methods. A large number of automated devices are now available. The accuracy of several of these has passed the rigorous performance criteria set by the British Hypertension Society. A good example is the Omron HEM 705 CP. In time the

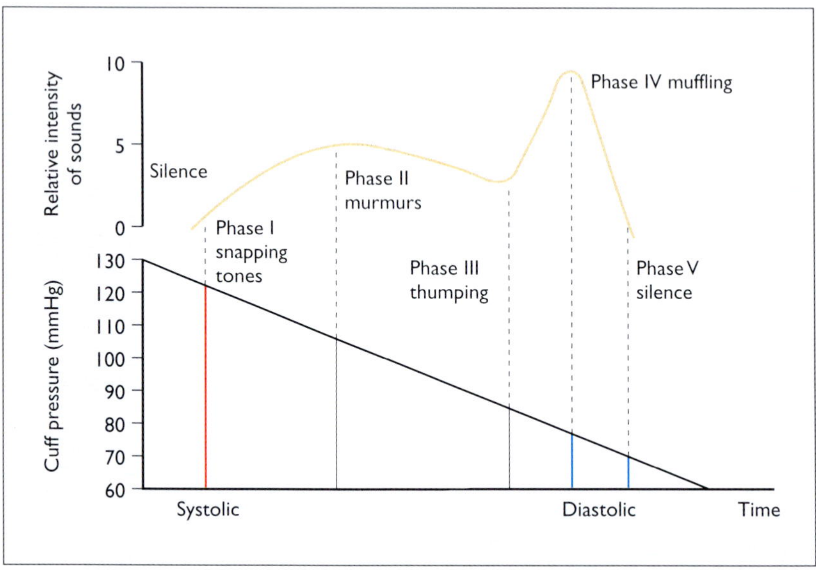

Figure 3.5. Change in Korotkoff sounds heard as cuff occlusion pressure is gradually lowered.

millimetre of mercury may be replaced by the 'kilopascal' as the unit of measurement. This may cause some consternation, but the switch to automated devices that are consistently accurate will at least remove much of the human observer variability [1].

The current mercury sphygmomanometer method has a number of clear-cut practical requirements to ensure optimum measurements – many of these will remain pertinent (Fig. 3.6). Sitting and standing measurements should be undertaken when there are symptoms of postural hypotension, when autonomic dysfunction might be expected (as in elderly or diabetic patients), when there may be circulatory volume depletion or in cases with secondary hypertension (see Chapter 10).

Given the wide degree of biological variation inherent in BP, it is perhaps surprising that casual BP measurements so strongly predict cardiovascular events. Some of the factors that influence this variability acutely are work, stress, mental and physical activity, alcohol intake

☐ Choose a bladder and cuff size appropiate to the dimensions of the arm:

Dimensions	Subject	Maximum arm circumference
13×4 cm	Small children	17 cm
18×8 cm	Medium sized children	26 cm
35×12.5 cm	Grown children and adults	42 cm

Accurate readings should be obtained in adults with arm circumferences greater than 42 cm by placing a cuff with a 35 cm bladder so that the centre of the bladder is over the brachial artery

☐ Ensure the patient is comfortably seated and rested for five minutes

☐ Remove tight or restrictive clothing

☐ Support the arm horizontally at the level of the heart

☐ If the measurement device employs a mercury column, place the manometer at eye level with the column vertical

☐ Estimate systolic pressure by palpating the brachial pulse and inflating the cuff until the pulsation disappears

☐ Reduce manometer pressure at 2 mmHg per second during auscultation

☐ Avoid digit preference by recording to the nearest 2 mmHg

☐ Note all measurements taken and, in addition, calculate an average value within a set time

☐ Make subsequent readings at the same time of day in relation to medication dosing

☐ Calibrate automatic monitors regularly

☐ Maintain and service equipment regularly

☐ Diastolic is recorded at phase V

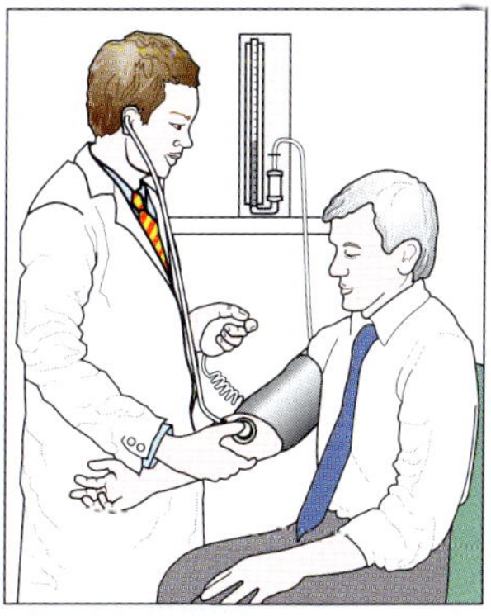

Figure 3.6. How to measure BP.

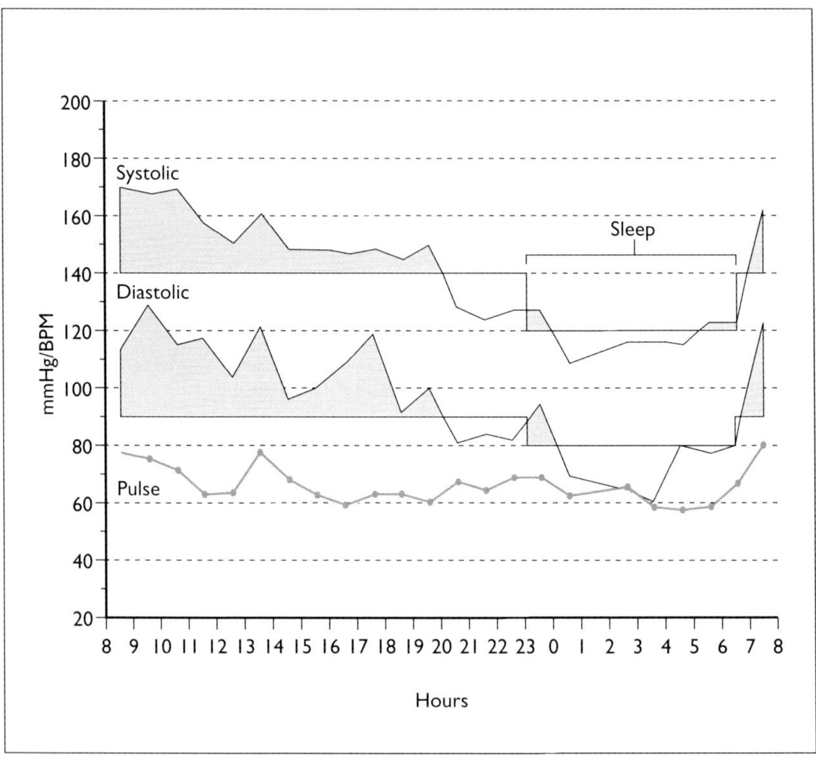

Figure 3.7. Example of ambulatory BP monitoring trace with normal nocturnal dip.

and smoking. Diurnal variability is also substantial, with an average fall in pressure of 20% during sleep (Fig. 3.7) – a fall that is blunted in the circumstance of secondary or accelerated hypertension. It is also important to recognize that initial BP levels characteristically fall progressively at sequential clinic or surgery visits. Consequently, it is generally sensible to take several sets of a series of at least three separated measurements before ascribing a diagnosis of hypertension (Table 3.1). The initial level of BP may determine the interval between sets of measurements. If levels are severe and obvious target organ damage is present there should be no delay in diagnosis and starting treatment.

Table 3.1. General guidelines for BP measurement

- Use recommendations from the British or American Hypertension Societies [2, 3]
- Measure routinely at least every 5 years in all adults until the age of 80 years
- Remeasure annually those with 'high–normal' values (135–139/85–89 mmHg)
- Make measurements in a consistent standardized fashion
- Use seated measurements routinely
- Measure sitting and standing in the elderly, diabetic or when symptoms indicate the need to detect postural hypotension
- Record both systolic and diastolic pressures
- Many adults require a large cuff (see Fig. 3.6)
- Measurement should begin after 5 minutes of rest
- Two or more readings separated by 2 minutes should be averaged; if the first two readings are markedly different, additional readings should be taken
- In mild uncomplicated hypertension paired readings at monthly intervals over 4 months should be used to guide treatment decisions
- BP should be evaluated together with other cardiovascular risk factors to determine overall risk (see Chapter 8)

Another important influence on measurement is that of the white-coat response (Fig. 3.8). This is a form of conditioned reflex that usually persists indefinitely without acclimatization. It is more marked in the presence of a doctor than a nurse, but there are no obvious characteristics of the patients who manifest this response [4]. It is not restricted to those who are obviously anxious in the clinical environment (see Chapter 10). A clue to this response may be found in a discrepancy between levels of measured BP and signs of target organ damage. Absence of target organ change when BP levels are very high suggests that these levels may not be sustained outside the clinic. Alternatively,

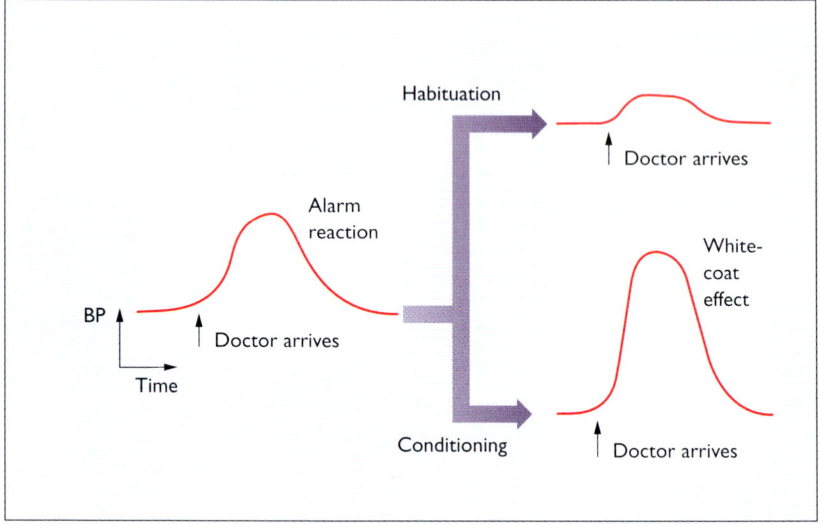

Figure 3.8. White-coat conditioned reflex in the consulting room.

such a discrepancy may alert the physician to other forms of transient or episodic hypertension that may be associated with conditions such as phaeochromocytoma or alcohol excess.

White-coat hypertension may best be defined as BP that is high in the clinic or surgery but significantly lower or normal at home or on 24-hour ambulatory BP monitoring (ABPM). The importance of this phenomenon is that it may be a significant influence in about 20% of people diagnosed as hypertensive in routine clinical practice – it is responsible for as many as half of the cases considered as 'resistant' [5]. Equally, it occurs to a greater or lesser extent in almost everybody – this means that values of BP recorded in different settings need to be adjusted to equate to the level that would be likely for that individual within the clinic (Table 3.2). This is an important issue, as our existing prognostic information with regard to BP is based upon a vast body of data from clinic measurements, and there is a danger that incorrect interpretation of home or ambulatory values leads to undertreatment. Table 3.2 also indicates that treatment

Table 3.2. Adjustment for interpretation of ABPM

Daytime average ambulatory BP monitoring	Adjustment factor (mmHg)	Clinic equivalent (mmHg)
148/83	12/7	160/90

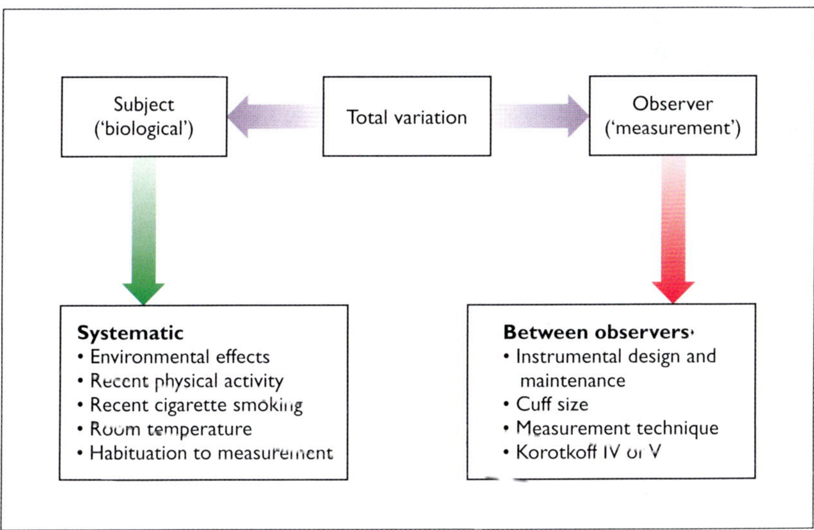

Figure 3.9. Summary of factors that influence the variability of BP.

decisions should be based on the adjusted average daytime BP rather than the average 24-hour BP.

It is also worth emphasizing that the white-coat response occurs on top of truly high BP in individuals who do have underlying hypertension and that the magnitude of the response is not affected by drug therapy.

Factors that influence the variability of BP are summarized in Figure 3.9.

Table 3.3. Indications for ABPM

- To determine usual BP in patients with borderline hypertension
- To identify and/or confirm white-coat hypertension
- To assess possible overtreatment in relation to symptoms
- To identify relation of BP levels to presumed side effects
- To assess BP diurnal variability in relation to severe or secondary hypertension
- To facilitate patient involvement in management

Much of the variability of BP measurement can be overcome by increasing the frequency of recording and removing it from the clinical setting. This can be achieved with self-operated devices that can be used at home and by 24-hour ABPM (see Fig. 3.7). There is good reason to believe that these methods will increasingly become standard practice in the clinical assessment and management of hypertension. Data from 24-hour ABPM show a much closer correlation with structural changes such as left ventricular hypertrophy than do casual measurements [6], but as yet the amount of follow-up data based on these techniques is limited [7]. Table 3.3 lists the circumstances in which ABPM may be particularly useful.

These recent refinements in measurement techniques will help to circumvent some of the uncertainties of interpretation, but BP is only one of several factors that contribute to overall cardiovascular risk. Regardless of the degree of repetition and accuracy with which a relatively modest BP level is recorded, many patients remain at high risk of cardiovascular events because of the combined effect of concurrent risk factors. Future refinement in 'cardiovascular' measurement needs to establish a composite parameter of the circulation that offers comprehensive predictive information. Left ventricular mass assessment offers a barometer of cumulative BP load akin to glycosylated haemoglobin in relation to diabetes, but left ventricular hypertrophy occurs relatively late in the hypertensive disease process. The familial, genetic and early life influences on future cardiovascular outcomes suggest that there are ways of detecting individuals at particular risk well in advance of rising BP or cardiac or vascular adaptations.

Chapter Summary

- Accurate and reliable measurement of BP is essential for both diagnosis of hypertension and in monitoring response to therapy.
- The mercury manometer is still widely used by the medical community, but may be replaced by automated devices and the kilopascal may become the unit of measurement in the future.
- Use a correctly sized cuff to avoid error. Where possible record the pressure under standardized and ideal conditions.
- Record both standing and sitting measurements when postural hypotension may be anticipated.
- Avoid potential errors in the use of the sphygmomanometer (e.g. inappropriate size of cuff or mercury manometer viewed from an incorrect angle).
- Consider whether or not the patient has white-coat hypertension.
- Consider whether ABPM may be useful.
- Consider the concurrent effects of other risk factors.

References

1. O'Brien E. Ave atque vale: the centenary of clinical sphygmomanometry. *Lancet* 1996; **348**: 1569–70.
2. Petrie JC, O'Brien ET, Littler WA, de Swiet M. Recommendations on blood pressure measurement. *Br Med J (Clin Restd)* 1986; **293**: 611–5.
3. American Society of Hypertension. Recommendations for routine blood pressure measurement by indirect cuff sphygmomanometry. *Am J Hypertens* 1992; **5**: 207–9.
4. Mancia G, Parati G, Pomidossi G, *et al.* Alerting reaction and rise in blood pressure during measurement by physician and nurse. *Hypertension* 1987; **9**: 209–15.
5. Pickering TG, James GD, Boddie C, *et al.* How common is white coat hypertension? *JAMA* 1988; **259**: 225–8.
6. Muiesan MML, Pasini GF, Salvetti M, *et al.* Cardiac and vascular structural changes, prevalence and relation to ambulatory blood pressure in a middle-aged population in northern Italy. *Hypertension* 1996; **27**: 1046–52.
7. Perloff D, Sokolow M, Cowan R. The prognostic value of ambulatory blood pressure in treated hypertensive patients. *J Hypertens* 1991; **9**(S1): S33–40.

chapter 4

Determinants of blood pressure and hypertension

BP is the principal focus of several homeostatic mechanisms within the circulation. Figure 4.1 illustrates the interacting factors that contribute to BP. Changes in any of these variables evoke powerful homeostatic secondary responses that tend to compensate for the directly evoked change while maintaining BP constant. In established hypertension the various feedback loops have adapted to operate at a higher level of BP. Evidence indicates that an abnormality can occur at every one of the steps in Figure 4.1. The problem of determining the cause of hypertension lies in interpreting the primacy of each of the identified 'abnormalities'. In each case the question is whether the change is causative or reactive to some other trigger upstream in the loop – and, if reactive, does the change represent an appropriate physiological adaptation or an inappropriate adaptation? For example, it seems highly likely that the upward resetting of baroreceptor sensitivity with developing hypertension occurs as a gradual adaptation rather than a primary defect. Structural changes within the walls of the small arteries might arise *de novo* as a primary causative abnormality, as an adaptive response to high BP or in response to an excessive neural or humoral signal.

BP is the product of cardiac output and peripheral resistance (Fig. 4.2). The small arteries (see Fig. 3.4) confer the major component of circulatory resistance, and as such their characteristics are so fundamental to the regulation of BP that it is tempting to seek the aetiology of hypertension here. Folkow suggested that a triggering pressor stimulus (e.g. noradrenaline [norepinephrine], angiotensin, endothelin, excess salt or any of numerous candidates) raises BP slightly and induces vascular hypertrophy or reorganization of the wall structure of the resistance arteries [1]. This rearrangement or change in conformation of the walls of the arteries acts to amplify the BP. It may be partly a response to a trophic effect of the initial stimulus and partly a mechanical adaptation to the rise in BP (Fig. 4.3) [2]. The key to this proposal is that a wide variety of initiating stimuli may lead to a slower progressive vascular amplification process. The final common path is a sustained increase in peripheral vascular resistance. The trigger may no longer be present or detectable by the time that hypertension becomes clinically established.

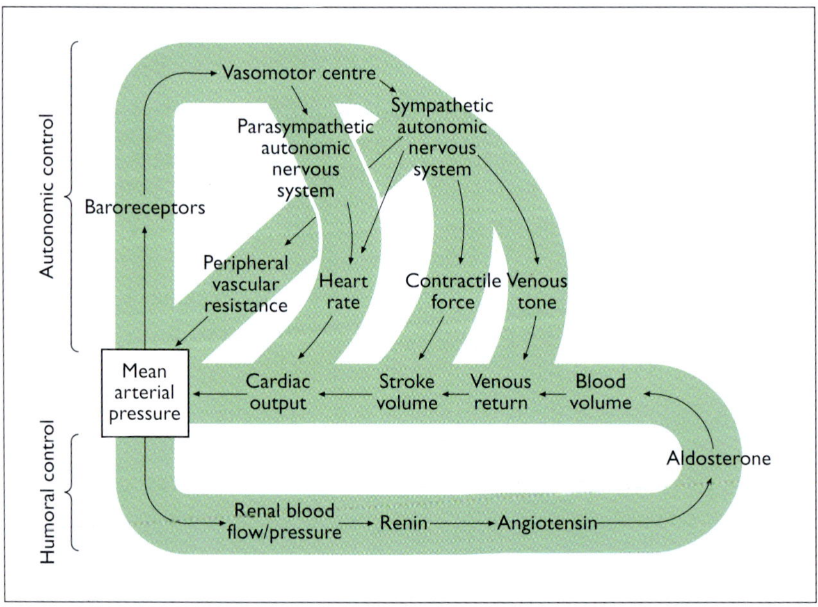

Figure 4.1. Interacting factors that contribute to BP.

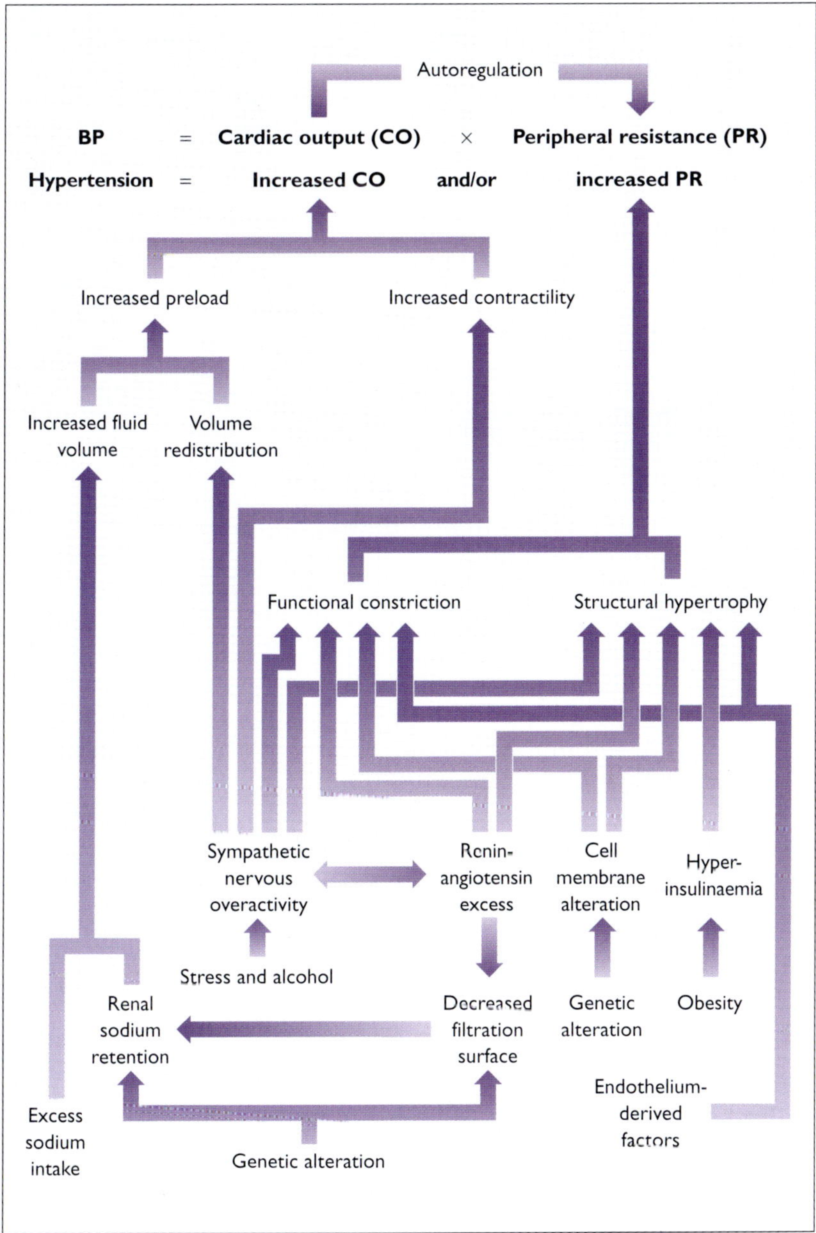

Figure 4.2. Hypertensive mechanisms.

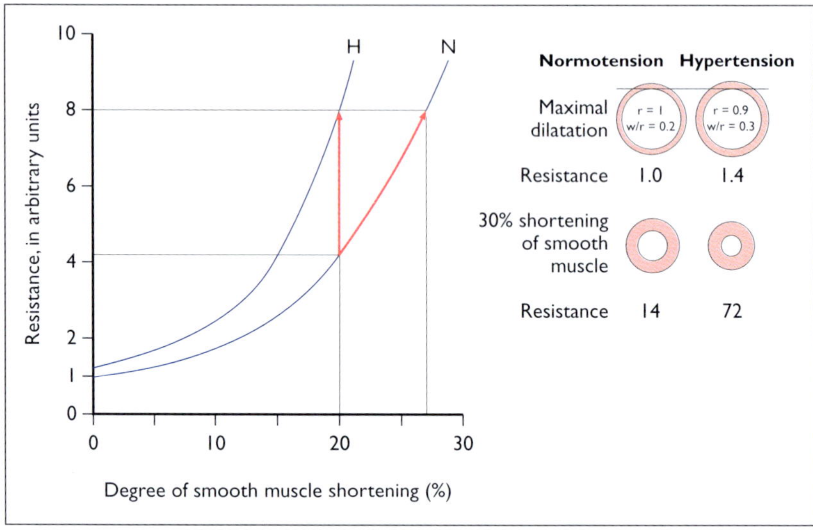

Figure 4.3. Impact of the structural change in hypertensive resistance arteries. 10% reduction of the inner radius (r) and an increase in the wall thickness (w) has increased the wall-to-lumen ratio (w/r) by 50% when the vessel is completely relaxed and dilated (right). The graph illustrates the haemodynamic consequences of the increase in w/r. Even at complete vascular relaxation the reistance to flow is elevated (1.0 versus 1.4 units). For equal degrees of vascular smooth muscle shortening the resistance is always higher in hypertension (H) than in normotension (N). (After Folkow [1]).

An alternative possibility is that the initiating defect may be the lack of a vasodilator mechanism within the vasculature rather than overactivity of a pressor mechanism – the net effect is the same. There is evidence for impairment of endothelial production of vasodilator nitric oxide associated with hypertension (Fig. 4.4) [3]. This endothelial abnormality has been demonstrated in the children of hypertensive parents at a stage while they themselves are still normotensive. A number of possible primary defects have been demonstrated in similar settings, but it remains very difficult to distinguish cause from consequence. Whatever the sequence it is accepted that once initiated vascular changes play an important role in maintaining high levels of BP – the mechanism involved is illustrated in Figure 4.5 [2].

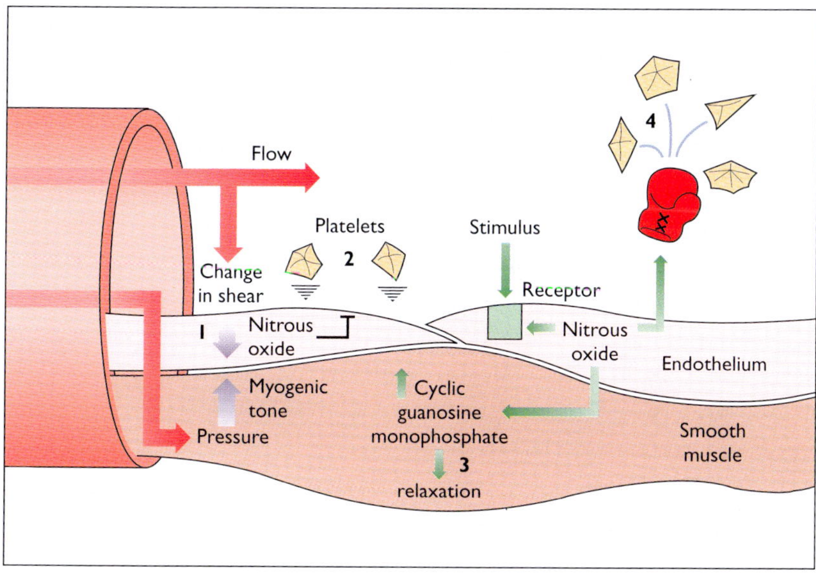

Figure 4.4. Endothelial autoregulation. 1. Counterbalance to the myogenic response in small vessels. 2. Inhibition of platelet adhesion. 3.Vascular smooth muscle relaxation. 4. Platelet disaggregation.

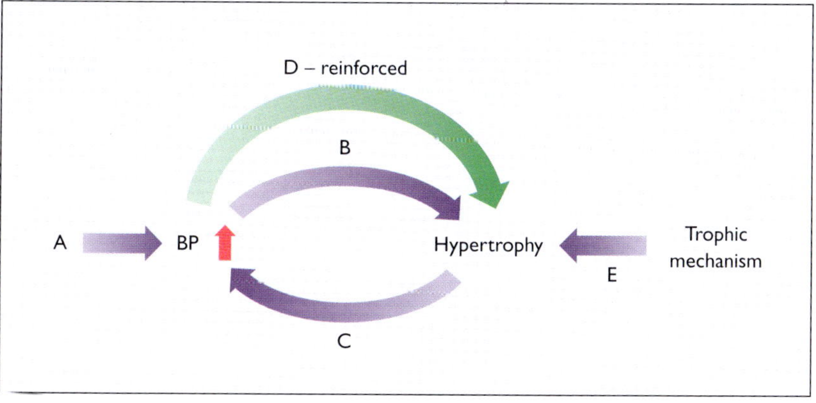

Figure 4.5. Pressor mechanisms in hypertension. Overactivity of a pressor mechanism A raises BP slightly, initiating positive feedback (via B and C) and a progressive rise in BP. Additional influences – D, a reinforced hypertrophic response to pressure, and, E, a direct hypertrophic agent – further enhance the pressor loop. (After Lever [1]).

There are many different viewpoints as to the nature of the key defect(s) in hypertension and several may concurrently be correct. Many current hypotheses are derived from research in animals – the relevance of these data to hypertension in humans must be interpreted with circumspection. The complexity of the control systems within the circulation indicates the numerous possibilities and the wide variety of secondary forms of hypertension with precisely defined mechanisms attests to the numerous ways of increasing BP (Table 4.1).

Although Table 4.1 lists some of the many forms of secondary hypertension for which the mechanisms are, to a greater or lesser degree, understood, more than 95% of all hypertension is of unknown cause and as such referred to as 'essential', 'idiopathic' or 'primary'.

In addition the variation in responsiveness to different antihypertensive medications among hypertensive patients indicates that different pathways may be active in different cases. This point is clearly seen among

Table 4.1. Some forms or associations of secondary hypertension for which the mechanisms are at least partly understood

Renal artery stenosis	1° Aldosteronism	Liquorice addiction
Pylelonephritis	Cushing's syndrome	Sympathomimetics
Obstructive nephropathy	Phaeochromocytoma	Chronic renal failure
	Vesico-ureteric reflux	Adrenal hyperplasia
Poliomyelitis	Porphyria	Renin JGA tumor
Gout	Acromegaly	Glomerulonephritis
Diabetes	Aortic coarctation	Polycystic kidneys
Amyloidosis	↑intracranial pressure	Systemic sclerosis
Carbenoxalone	Oral contraceptive	Haemolytic-uremic syndrome
MAO-inhibitors	Endothelinoma	
Pre-eclampsia	Lead poisoning	
Alcohol	Corticosteroids	

black African or African–Caribbean hypertensive patients, who are typically less responsive to β-blockers and angiotensin-converting enzyme (ACE) inhibitors [4]. This characteristic probably relates to relatively low plasma renin levels, which indicates that hypertension in blacks is not driven by activation of the renin–angiotensin system. Similar variations exist within ethnic groups and clues to the expression of different genotypes may lie in varying sensitivities to different therapies. While rare forms of hypertension (such as those associated with hyperaldosteronism) are related to a single gene defect, it seems clear that the bulk of 'essential' hypertension arises from multiple contributing factors. Variation in BP levels within a given population may partly be explained by the combined effects of multiple genes.

The familial aggregation of BP emphasizes the importance of an inheritable component of essential hypertension. The strength of this component must be considered in the context of the shared family environment. Estimates of the genetic contribution to the variability of BP vary from 25% in family studies to 75% in twin studies. The latter may, in part at least, be more correctly attributed to the influence of a shared intrauterine environment. The associations between early developmental characteristics, future emergence of cardiovascular risk factors and ultimately cardiovascular events may be explained by fetal programming through variations in the intrauterine environment or maternal nutrition, but again it is difficult to prioritize the environmental or genetic influence (Fig. 4.6) [5].

Environmental or dietary factors

A large number of environmental factors are regarded as possible determinants of BP. Table 4.2 includes a variety of factors for which the evidence supporting a relationship with hypertension ranges from circumstantial or weak to strong and probably causative. For instance a number of surveys suggest a link between calcium intake and BP, but the evidence is inconsistent, unsupported by meta-analysis and

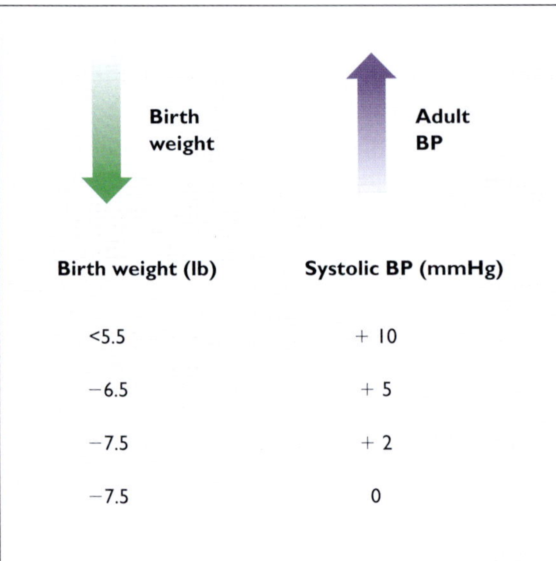

Figure 4.6. Relationship of birth weight with adult BP levels.

Table 4.2. Environmental factors associated with hypertension

- Excess sodium salt intake
- Lack of physical activity
- Overweight
- Insufficient dietary fibre
- Magnesium deficiency
- Excess saturated fats
- Stress
- Alcohol excess
- Low dietary potassium
- Coffee
- Low dietary calcium
- Low vitamin C intake
- Lead exposure

insufficient to recommend increasing dietary calcium to either treat or prevent hypertension. Several components of a vegetarian diet may contribute to lower BP – among these are increased potassium, fibre and vitamin C. There is good evidence for low levels of dietary potassium

Table 4.3. Estimated diet of late Palaeolithic humans versus that of contemporary North Americans [7]

Nutrient	Palaeolithic diet (assuming 35% meat)	Current North American diet
■ Total energy		
protein (%)	30	12
carbohydrate (%)	45–50	46
fat (%)	20–25	42
■ Polyunsaturated:saturated fat ratio	1.41	0.44
■ Fibre (g/day)	86	10–20
■ Sodium (mg)	604	3400
■ Potassium (mg)	6790	2400
■ Potassium:sodium ratio	12:1	0.7:1
■ Calcium (mg)	1520	740

being involved in hypertension, and in addition low potassium intake is associated with an increased risk of stroke – an association that appears partly independent of BP. Potassium depletion increases BP and potassium supplementation is effective in lowering BP, even in 'normotensive' individuals [6] (see Chapter 8 for the protective effect of potassium against BP and stroke). The changes in the nature of our diet from that of our ancestors may hold important clues to the aetiology of hypertension (Table 4.3) [7].

Salt, kidneys and BP

Of all the dietary or environmental factors that may influence BP some of the strongest evidence exists for the causative role of dietary sodium. The early writings of the Chinese Yellow Emperor noted that salt in the diet led to hardening of the pulse (Fig. 4.7). Salt intake in westernized communities may have changed more than any other dietary

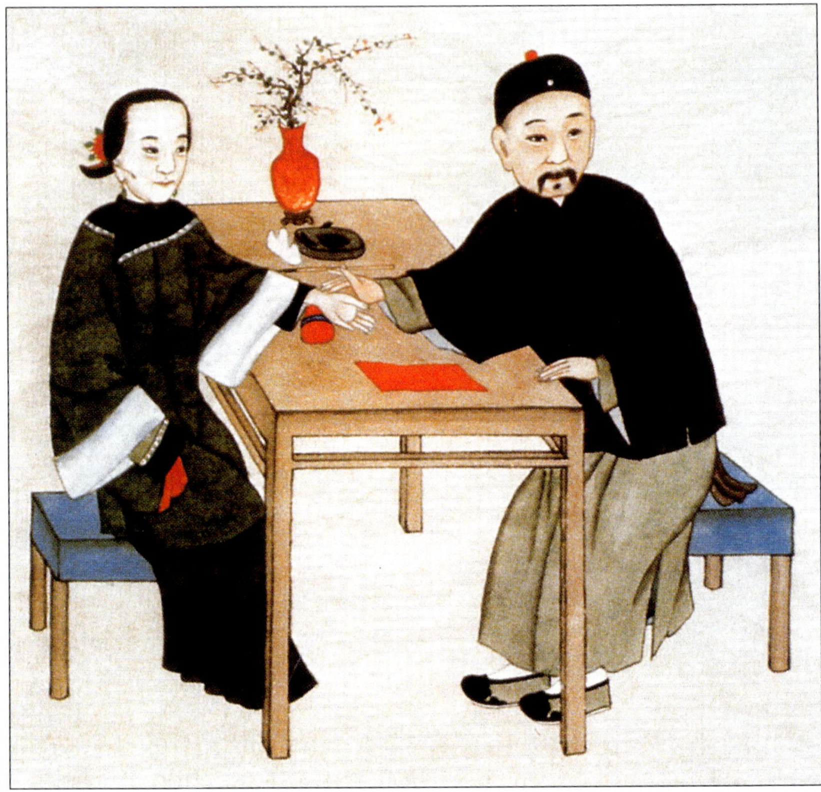

Figure 4.7. An early painting of a Chinese physician feeling radial pulse and recognizing the association between high salt intake and hardening of the pulse.

component, even in recent times, and is greatly in excess of that required. This has followed patterns of food preservation and processing driven by taste and the food industry. All communities or cultures that do not have essential hypertension and in which BP does not rise with age also have low salt intake [8]. For example, the Yanomamö Indians in Brazil excrete only about 2 mmol of sodium per day, which reflects a very low dietary intake, and they have an average adult BP of 103/65 mmHg (Fig. 1.4). The direct relationship between dietary salt intake and BP has sometimes proved difficult to detect within some western populations because the customary salt intake is so high that too few individuals have a low enough intake to build the whole picture. However, a review which summarizes the results of 21 between-population studies and 14 within-population studies showed that, in keeping with trial evidence (see Chapter 8), the relationship between salt and BP was larger than generally appreciated and increased with age [9].

An overview of these observational data indicates a linear relationship between salt intake and BP, such that a 100 mmol increment in dietary sodium is associated with a 6 mmHg rise in systolic BP (1 teaspoon salt = almost 150 mmol of sodium).

There are a number of proposed mechanisms whereby sodium may elevate BP (Table 4.4). Among these the idea that accumulation of salt and water within the walls of the resistance arteries – effectively waterlogging the walls – may be a priming mechanism that leads directly to the structural impact described in Figure 4.3. More likely is the concept that excess sodium pushes cellular sodium–calcium exchange within vascular smooth muscle towards higher levels of intracellular calcium. This may be the initial pressor trigger (A) described in Figure 4.5.

Not everyone responds to sodium in the same way. Susceptibility may be related to a particular sensitivity of vascular smooth muscle to sodium or to an abnormality in renal sodium handling. Both these circumstances may be caused by a defect in a similar cellular ion pump – in vascular smooth muscle, leading to increased intracellular calcium, and in the kidney, leading to an inability to excrete sodium. Another possibility that

Table 4.4. Possible mechanisms of sodium causing hypertension

- Increased circulatory volume
- Increased intracellular calcium
- Thickening of vessel walls
- Enhanced sympathetic activity
- Enhanced potassium and calcium excretion
- Increased insulin resistance

has been proposed is that the population of nephrons within hypertensive kidneys is either numerically reduced or functionally compromised. Reduced nephron number is a possible mechanism whereby impaired fetal growth and, hence, low birth weight are associated with increased BP in adult life. Again, reduced nephron number or function impairs the ability to excrete sodium. The normal kidney contributes powerfully to volume and pressure regulation by operating within a tight relationship of 'pressure–natriuresis' – a small change in pressure causes a large change in water and sodium excretion. This homeostatic mechanism may be shifted upwards in hypertension [10].

The view that the cause of essential hypertension lies within the kidney is supported by the varieties of renal parenchymal disease that are associated with hypertension – perhaps starting with Bright's observation, over 100 years ago, of shrunken kidneys linked with arterial thickening and vascular catastrophes. Transplantation studies in animals have shown that hypertension follows the kidney – that is, recipients of a kidney from a hypertensive animal develop hypertension and hypertensive recipients of a kidney from a normotensive animal become normotensive. The same phenomenon of hypertension developing in human recipients of kidneys transplanted from hypertensive donors has also been described.

Physical inactivity

There is a close relationship between level of physical activity and BP (Fig. 4.8). Among men and women, sedentary normotensive individuals have a 20–50% greater risk of becoming hypertensive than their more active, physically fitter peers. Diminishing physical activity is another trait that follows 'westernization' of lifestyle. Maintaining even a modest level of regular physical activity protects against the development of hypertension and diabetes, and also against the development or progression of most other cardiovascular risk factors. Beyond this, increased exercise and physical fitness protect against both heart attack and stroke, and prospective studies have shown increased survival over long-term follow-up.

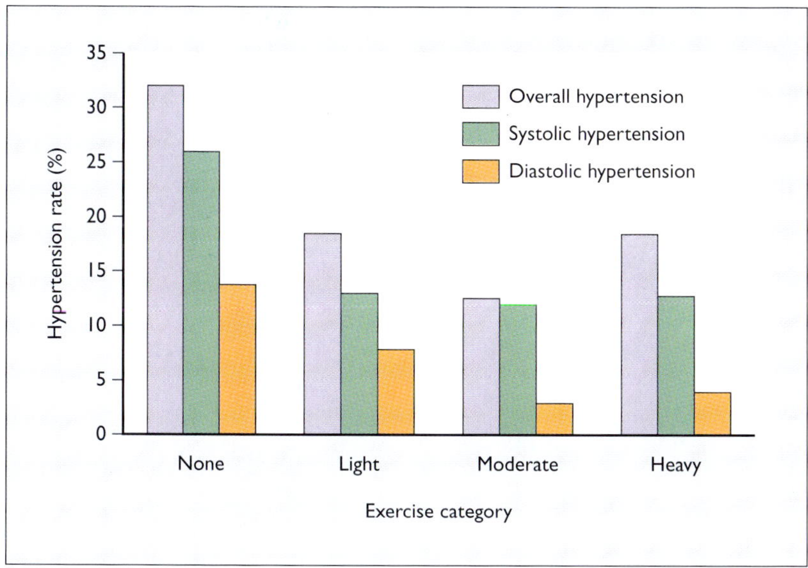

Figure 4.8. Hypertension is more prevalent among women with lower levels of physical activity. Adapted from Reaven [11].

'Physical activity' should not be confused with 'exercise', which usually denotes some form of sport that requires particular preparation or equipment. Rather, physical activity refers to expenditure of energy through the tasks of daily living – activity that is minimized by the burgeoning gadgets of the late twentieth century.

The mechanisms whereby physical activity influences BP are listed in Table 4.5. The corollary is that physical inactivity may cause hypertension.

Obesity

Obesity, hypertension and diabetes overlap to a considerable extent among communities in which any of the three conditions are prevalent (see Chapter 6). The common thread may be a genetic overlap or a shared determinant in aetiology, such as physical inactivity. Certainly,

Table 4.5. Mechanisms whereby physical exercise influences BP

Increased physical activity causes:	
Increased	**Decreased**
■ Endothelial nitric oxide production	■ Total peripheral resistance
■ Insulin sensitivity	■ Noradrenaline spillover
■ Oxygen uptake	■ Resting pulse

the temporal trends of the conditions emerging in western communities over the past century track with diminishing physical activity, in an interval far too brief to expect any change in the gene pool.

Hypertension is evidently closely associated with obesity, but is obesity an independent risk factor for hypertension? There are several possible

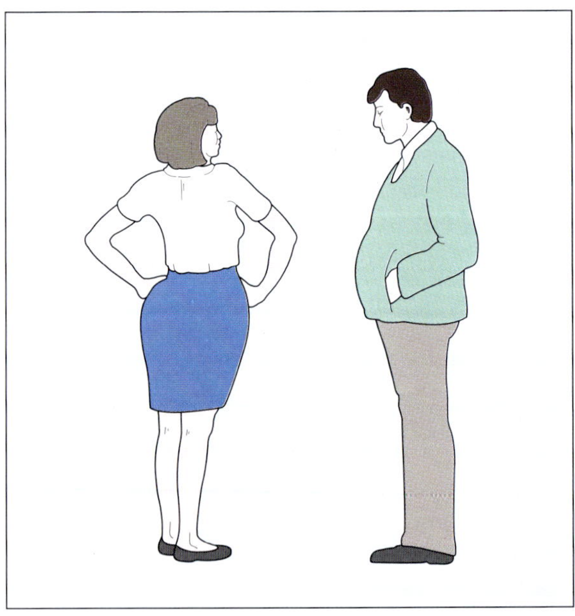

Figure 4.9. Patterns of fat distribution: the typical android central distribution with a 'pot-belly' represents an important risk factor, whereas a slim waist with large hips – more typically female – is relatively advantageous.

Table 4.6. Mechanisms whereby obesity increases blood pressure

- Increased sympathetic activation
- Increased insulin resistance (see Chapter 6)
- Mechanical contribution to increased peripheral vascular resistance

'confounders' in this relationship – dietary factors, including salt and fat, physical activity level and measurement bias in patients with large upper arms. Furthermore, increasing levels of overweight are associated with increasing levels of a cluster of other risk factors for cardiovascular disease (Fig. 9.3). Body mass index (BMI) is a poor marker of obesity – a performance athlete can have the same BMI as a podgy couch potato. Nevertheless, various markers of obesity, including BMI, do suggest that overweight is associated with higher BP levels. The mechanisms whereby obesity might cause or contribute to hypertension are listed in Table 4.6.

The causal association with hypertension becomes stronger with an index of 'central obesity', such as 'waist:hip ratio'. This is also closely linked to metabolic features of the insulin-resistance syndrome and emphasizes the importance of patterns of fat distribution (Fig. 4.9). Paradoxically it has been suggested that lean hypertensives have a worse cardiovascular prognosis than those who are overweight with apparently equivalent brachial BPs. In part, this may be attributable to the necessary, but imprecise, adjustment in cuff size needed to measure BP in individuals with larger arms. An under-sized cuff results in an overestimate of the real BP.

Alcohol

The dose response between alcohol intake and increased BP levels is striking (Fig. 4.10) [12]. The hypertensive response to alcohol takes several days to settle after withdrawal. Nationally, at least in the UK, BPs are higher on Mondays than Thursdays – reflecting the common pattern of binge drinking at weekends. This pattern may not pertain

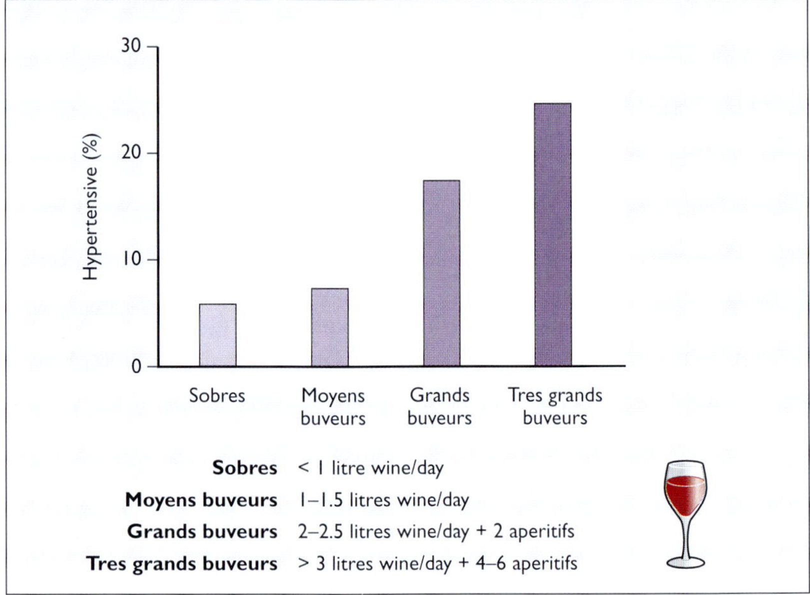

Figure 4.10. Prevalence of hypertension (>150/90 mmHg) among French soldiers in 1915 according to habitual alcohol intake. Adapted from Lian [12].

in France, where there appears to be a more steady state of alcohol consumption. As much as 10% of hypertension in men may relate to alcohol excess, and may explain the resistance to therapy among some hypertensive cases that are difficult to control with multiple drugs. Assessment of alcohol consumption is therefore an important part of the history and clinical examination.

In contrast to the acute vasodilator effect of alcohol in the skin, small arteries in the skeletal muscle circulation show a pressor response. Alcohol stimulates sympathetic activity and, in the extreme case, may present as a pseudophaeochromocytoma syndrome. Another alcohol-induced endocrine problem is that of pseudo-Cushing's syndrome. In both these settings the clinical pictures (including non-dipping refractory hypertension) and the biochemical indices (including raised catecholamines or cortisol) mimic the eponymous conditions until alcohol is withdrawn.

High alcohol intake is also associated with cigarette smoking, and new evidence shows that among men heavy smokers tend to have higher BP than do non-smokers.

Interacting genotypes and phenotypes: genes and environment

The genetic 'mosaic' in Figure 4.11 illustrates how environmental factors may amplify the expression of particular theoretical genotypes with resultant hypertension. Again, reference to black African populations illustrates the potential impact of gene plus environment interactions. Among people living in the UK, higher levels of BP are recognized in those of African descent than in Caucasians. However, the prevalence of hypertension is extremely low in parts of rural Africa. The implication is that the building blocks for hypertension are innately present and that 'westernization' leads to expression of the condition. Migration studies within Africa that tracked those who moved from rural to urban environments indicate that BP rises abruptly on arrival in the city. The most likely 'urban' contributing factors are weight gain and increased sodium intake, decreased potassium intake and raised pulse rates, which presumably reflect increased stress [13] This issue is further illustrated by the comparison of the relationship between age and BP in westernized and 'unacculturated' societies (Fig. 1.3 and 1.4). A progressive rise of BP with age is inappropriately accepted as the biological norm in western communities. In 'unacculturated' populations, BP remains steady throughout adult life – hypertension is not a feature of such populations. The important differences between the two lie in lifestyles rather than in genes.

Identification of the genes involved in hypertension will enhance our understanding of the pathogenesis and may also serve to characterize those patients who will respond either beneficially or adversely to particular therapies. However, even complete gene mapping is unlikely to lead to a magic therapeutic solution and attention to environmental factors through a population-based approach will remain of prime importance.

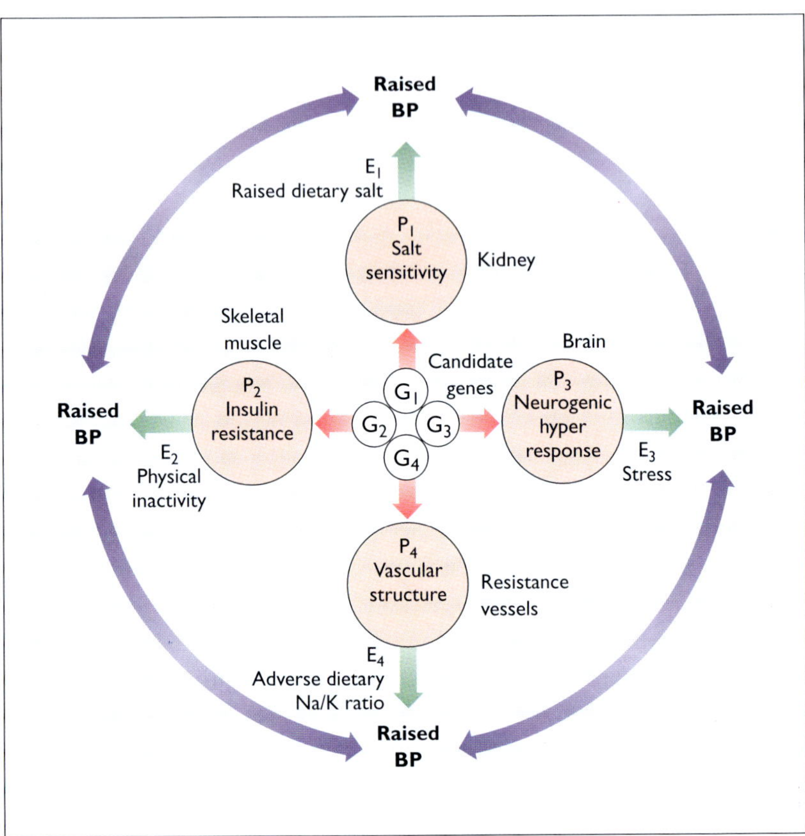

Figure 4.11. A variety of different genotypes (G) leads to different phenotypic (P) expression. These are subject to various environmental (E) influences producing high BP by different pathways.

CHAPTER SUMMARY

- The pathogenesis of essential hypertension is multifactorial.
- Variation in BP levels within a given population may be partly explained by the combined effects of multiple genes and the environment.
- Familial aggregation of BP emphasizes the importance of an inheritable component of essential hypertension and/or shared environment.
- Changes in the nature of our diet from that of our ancestors may hold important clues to the aetiology of hypertension.
- There is a close relationship between the level of physical activity and BP.
- Obesity, hypertension and diabetes overlap to a considerable extent among communities in which the three conditions are prevalent.
- For the PHCT there are four key modifiable areas: excess intake of calories (obesity), salt and alcohol and inadequate exercise.
- Identification of the genes involved in hypertension will enhance the understanding of the pathogenesis, but attention to environmental factors through a population-based approach will remain of primary importance.

REFERENCES

1. Folkow B. Structural factor in primary and secondary hypertension. *Hypertension* 1990; **16**: 89–101.
2. Lever AF. Slow pressor mechanisms in hypertension: a role for hypertrophy of resistance vessels? *J Hypertens* 1986; **4**: 515–24.
3. Panza JA, Quyumi AA, Brush JE, *et al.* Abnormal endothelium-dependant vascular relaxation in patients with essential hypertension. *N Engl J Med* 1990; **323**: 22–7.
4. Materson BJ, Reda DJ, Cushman WC. Department of Veterans Affairs single-drug therapy of hypertension study. *Am J Hypertens* 1995; **8**: 189–92.
5. Barker DJP. Fetal origins of coronary heart disease. *BMJ* 1995; **311**: 171–4.
6. Khaw KT, Thom S. Randomised double-blind crossover trial of potassium on blood pressure in normal subjects. *Lancet* 1982; **ii**: 1127–9.
7. Eaton SB, Eaton S, Konner SJ, *et al.* An evolutionary perspective enhances understanding of human nutritional requirements. *J Nutr* 1996; **126**: 1732–40.
8. Dahl LK. Salt and hypertension. *Am J Clin Nutr* 1972; **25**: 231–44.
9. Law MR, Frost CD, Wald NJ. Analysis of data from trials of salt reduction. *Br Med J* 1991; **302**: 819–24.
10. Guyton AC. Physiologic regulation of arterial pressure. *Am J Cardiol* 1961; **8**: 401–7.
11. Reaven PD, Barrett-Connor E, Edelstein S. Relation between leisure-time physical activity and blood pressure in older women. *Circulation* 1991; **83**: 559–65.
12. Lian C. L'alcoolisme, cause d'hypertension arterielle. *Bull Acad Med* 1915; **74**: 525–8.
13. Poulter N, Khaw KT, Hopwood BEC *et al.* The Kenyan Luo migration study: observations on the initiation of a rise in blood pressure. *BMJ* 1990; **300**: 967–72.

chapter 5

Natural history

Increasing levels of either an elevated systolic or an elevated diastolic BP increase the risk of death (Table 5.1) [1]. Contrary to the emphasis historically placed on diastolic pressure, systolic pressure is a better predictor of subsequent cardiovascular disease than is diastolic pressure (Fig. 5.1) [1]. For this reason, allied with the trial evidence for the benefits of treating isolated systolic BP (Chapter 12), it is inappropriate to ignore systolic pressure and thresholds for intervention should be based on either elevated systolic or diastolic pressures.

Table 5.1. Multiple Risk Factor Intervention Trial 'screenees': systolic pressure and age-adjusted all-cause mortality at 10 years*

Systolic BP (mmHg) stratum	Death rate/1000	Relative risk	Excess deaths (%)
<110	32.1	1.0	0.0
110–119	34.6	1.1	3.4
120–129	38.0	1.2	12.0
130–139	45.9	1.4	22.5
140–149	55.2	1.7	21.1
150–159	73.2	2.3	18.1
160–169	**82.0**	**2.6**	**9.5**
170–179	**106.1**	**3.3**	**6.1**
≥180	**142.8**	**4.4**	**7.3**

*Bold entries are the 'high-risk' group.

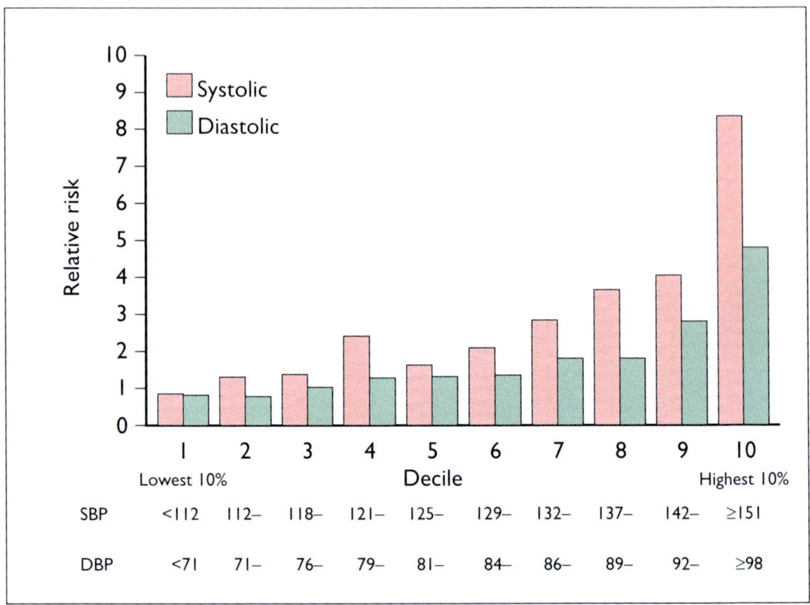

Figure 5.1. Adjusted relative risk of stroke death according to deciles of baseline systolic blood pressure (SBP) and diastolic blood pressure (DBP) in 347 978 men screened for Multiple Risk Factor Intervention Trial.

Whilst on average in westernized populations systolic BP rises across the whole age range, diastolic BP peaks in the sixth decade and then declines, thereby producing an increased pulse pressure (SBP-DBP). This is the result of large arteries becoming increasingly stiff and less compliant with age. It is therefore not suprising that studies have shown that a wide pulse pressure which results from arterial disease, at least in those aged over 50 years, is a better predictor of adverse cardiovascular events than either raised systolic or diastolic BP alone.

The macrovascular complications of hypertension are mainly produced by atherosclerotic, thrombotic and haemorrhagic vascular disease (Fig. 5.2).

The vast majority of excess deaths attributable to raised BP are due to coronary heart disease (CHD), stroke, heart failure and renal failure. In the UK and other parts of the western world, the major

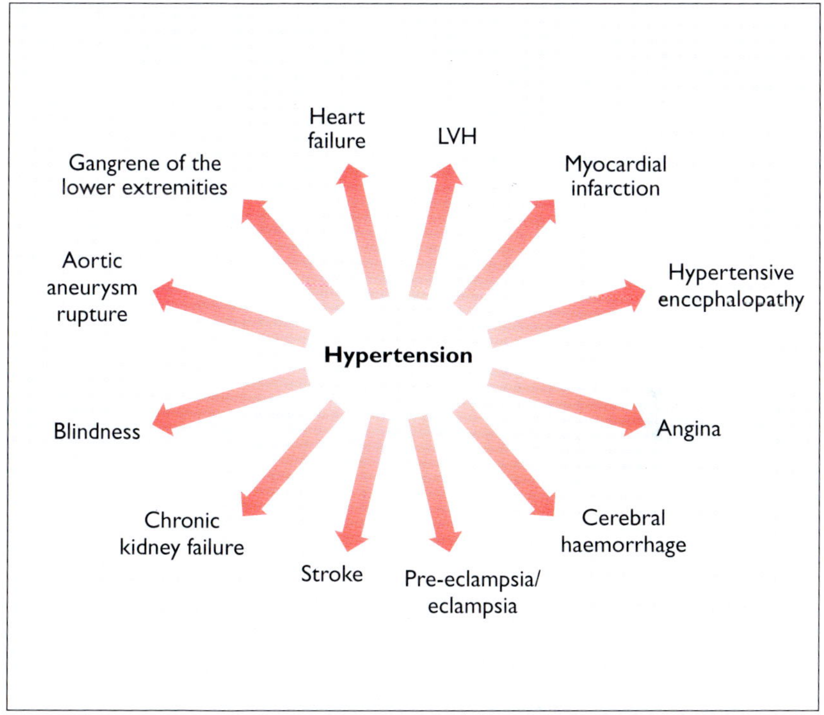

Figure 5.2. Diseases attributable to hypertension.

current causes of death associated with elevated BP are CHD and stroke, although earlier in the twentieth century renal failure was proportionally more important. As the population ages and prevention and treatment of hypertension improves, heart failure is increasing as a major adverse effect and is one of the main causes of hospital admission for the elderly [2]. It is important to note that in the UK and most of the western industrialized world, although not in other parts of the world, 3–4 CHD events occur for each stroke event attributable to raised BP (Fig. 5.3) [3]. These variable ratios presumably reflect that other risk factors interact differentially with raised BP to produce stroke and CHD. This highlights the fact that, although the two disorders share common risk factors, these risk factors are not

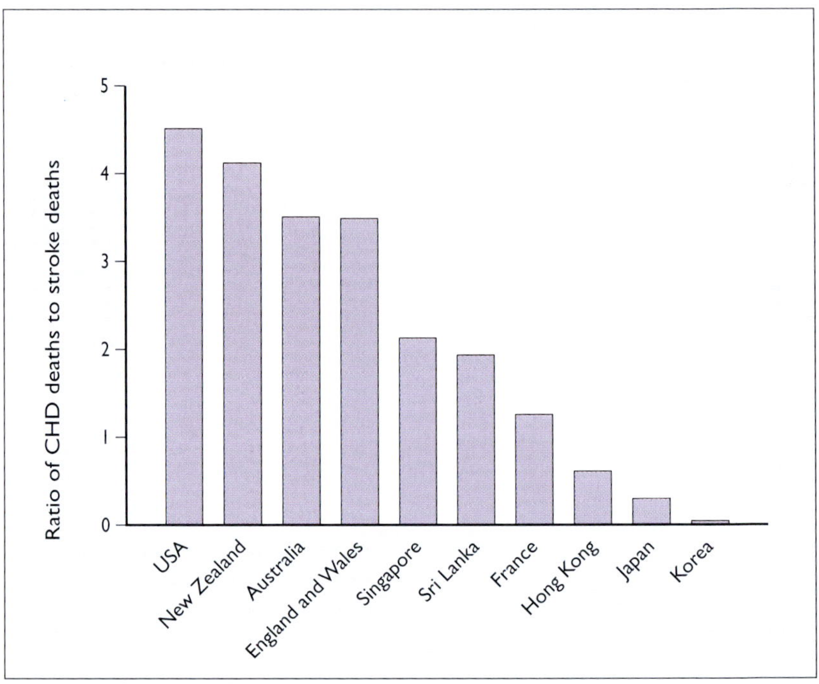

Figure 5.3. Number of deaths as a result of CHD for each cerebrovascular death in men, 1985–1989 [3].

of equal importance for the two conditions. Raised BP is the major risk factor for stroke [4], whereas abnormal lipids are the key determinant for CHD [5]. The large proportion of stroke events compared with CHD events in the Veterans' Administration study (Fig. 5.4) [6] reflects the high levels of BP of those people included. Figure 5.4 also shows how the profile of risks associated with hypertension has changed since the introduction of effective antihypertensive agents.

The risk of stroke and CHD events associated with increasing BP levels is shown in Figure 1.2 [7]. These data highlight the fact that there is no threshold below which BP is 'safe' and that a cut-off point for the definition of 'hypertension' on the basis of future risk can be made only on an arbitrary basis. The continous nature of this relationship also has major implications for preventive strategy (Chapter 8). Nevertheless, the

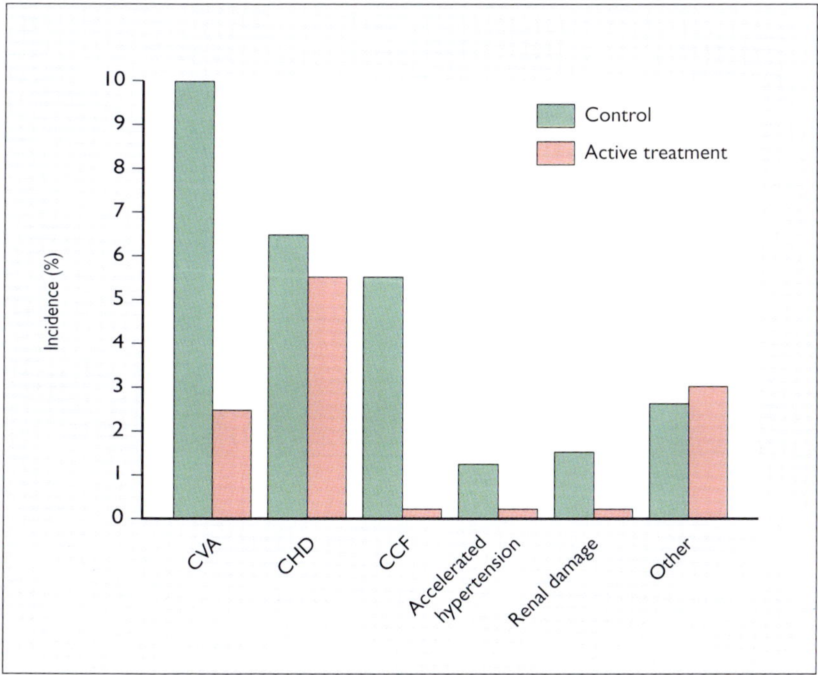

Figure 5.4. Stroke events compared with coronary heart disease and other events in a study by the Veterans Administration.

majority of strokes and heart attacks attributed to BP occur in people who are conventionally considered 'normotensive' (see Table 5.1).

Hypertension is commonly associated with some degree of renal impairment. In cases of severe essential hypertension, vascular changes within the kidney lead to nephrosclerosis and impairment of renal function. Prior to the introduction of antihypertensive therapy, this resulted in irreversible renal failure. Fortunately, effective antihypertensive treatment now usually prevents the progression of renal disease. Hypertension may, on the other hand, be caused by a primary renal or renovascular pathology, which in some circumstances responds to curative treatment (e.g. angioplasty or surgery for renal artery stenosis).

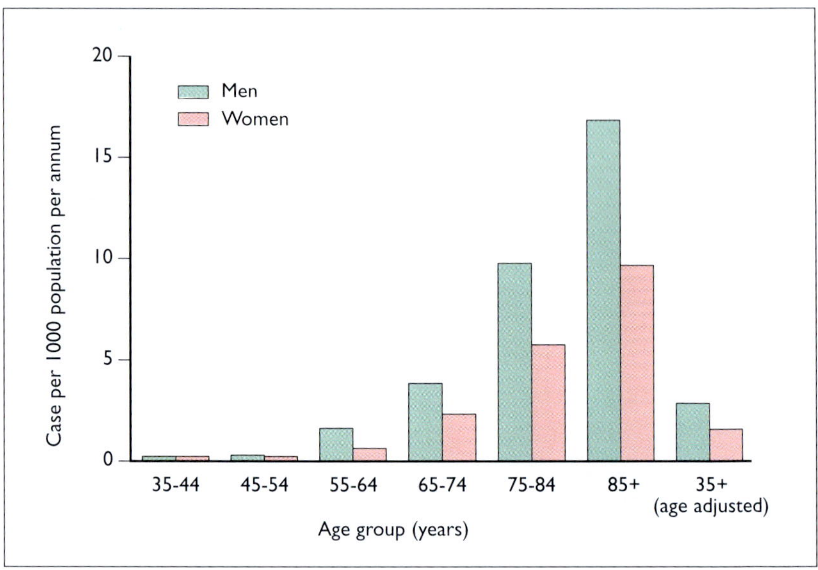

Figure 5.5. Incidence of cardiac failure in a UK population (Hillingdon Heart Failure Study, U.K).

As discussed elsewhere in this book (see Chapter 6), hypertension and diabetes are commonly associated; in this group of patients progressive deterioration in renal function is commonly encountered. Good BP control is very important in patients with progressive renal disease of any kind [8], as emphasized by the drastically diminished survival of haemodialysis patients whose hypertension is inadequately treated.

Although cardiac failure may occur as a consequence of long-standing, untreated hypertension (as reflected in Fig. 5.4), it is now increasing because of the changing demography of the population and the success of other preventive interventions (Fig. 5.5). Cardiac failure is often preceded by hypertension [9], but atherosclerotic CHD is probably an equally important contributing factor. The relationship here is somewhat circular, as hypertension is itself an important risk factor for coronary atherosclerosis. When hypertension is associated with cardiac failure, the resultant morbidity and mortality rates are high (Fig. 5.6).

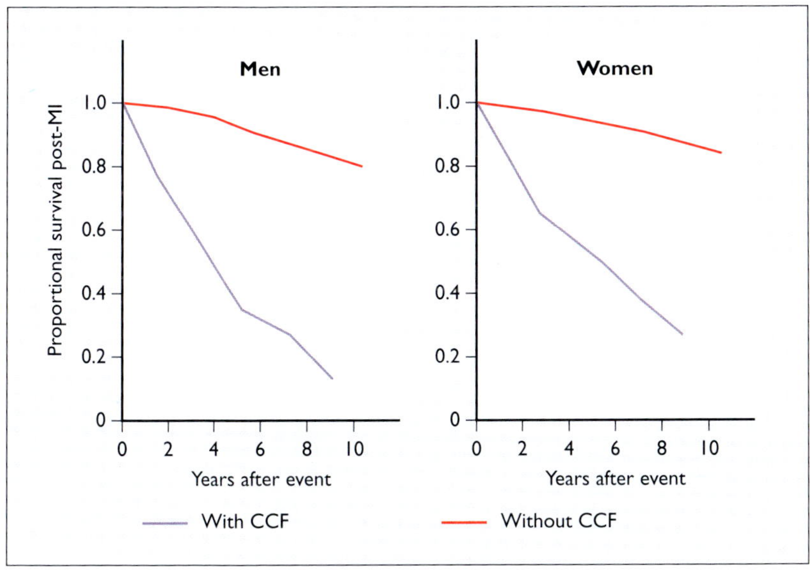

Figure 5.6. Survival following MI with and without congestive cardiac failure in men and women at age 45 years or over.

Hypertension is also the major cause of left ventricular hypertrophy (LVH). The classic cardiac adaptation to sustained hypertension is concentric left ventricular (LV) hypertrophy. This consists of LV wall thickening, as well as an increased LV mass index. However, it has been observed that other forms of cardiac adaptation are also common. The LV geometry may be normal; alternatively, the walls may be thick with no increase in LV mass index (called concentric remodelling). Finally, the LV cavity may be dilated, which results in an increased LV mass index even though the walls remain a normal size (termed eccentric hypertrophy). Compared with normotensive patients, those with hypertension have a high risk of sudden death, which may be related to the increased prevalence of frequent and complex ventricular arrhythmias that have been observed. Both ventricular arrhythmias and sudden death are particularly common in hypertensive patients with LVH as compared with those without. An independent risk

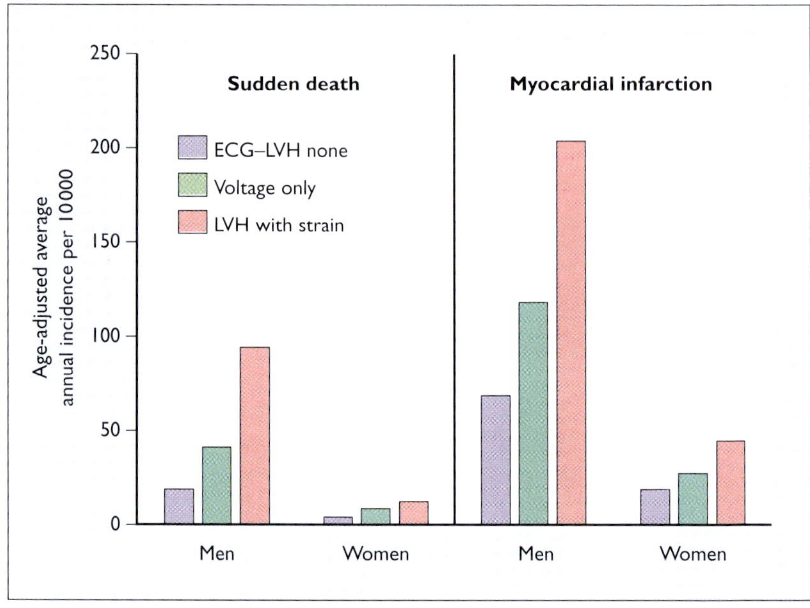

Figure 5.7. Sudden death, myocardial infarction and LVH in men and women.

factor for CHD death, LVH is associated with increased rates of sudden death, presumably because of arrhythmias (Fig. 5.7) [10].

Obesity and diabetes are also independent causes of LVH and hence, given the frequent coexistence of hypertension with these other two conditions, LVH is commonly found in hypertensive patients. Although LVH can be detected using ECG and/or chest radiography (increased cardiothoracic ratio), these are insensitive tests for LVH. When LVH is apparent on routine ECG or chest radiography there is usually a marked degree of LVH, and therefore its detection in this way is associated with a significantly worsened cardiovascular prognosis.

More sensitive, but more expensive, for detecting LVH is the echocardiograph. This is a helpful and certainly cost-effective tool in differentiating white-coat from 'real' hypertension.

All the adverse consequences of hypertension detailed in Figure 5.2 are related in some way to problems in the blood vessels – for the most part either occlusion of the arteries (by accumulating atheromatous plaque and thrombosis) or rupture of the arteries. Structural changes in the vasculature in association with elevated BP have been recognized since Bright described thickening of the aortic wall and left ventricle in patients who suffered hypertensive renal disease. Nevertheless, the question remains as to whether the structural changes associated with hypertension are primary and drive, to some extent, the rise in BP, or adaptive – a troublesome consequence of the raised BP. Why the structural changes in blood vessels should be troublesome in humans is not entirely clear, but it is obvious that when 'adaptive' vascular changes progress to atherosclerosis the situation is highly abnormal. By contrast, in the giraffe BP levels in excess of 300 mmHg are associated with profound arterial hypertrophy, while seemingly carrying no increased risk of cardiovascular disease [11]. However, it is clear that raised BP in humans is associated with a complex pattern of structural changes in the cardiovascular system. These structural changes include:

- Cardiac hypertrophy
- Thickening of the walls of large elastic and muscular arteries
- Remodelling of small muscular arteries, which results in increased wall-to-lumen ratio (Fig. 4.3)
- Reduced number of vessels in the microcirculation
- Lengthening of small arteries.

It may be that some aspects of these changes are associated with the initiating process of hypertension, and that others develop as adaptations to the haemodynamic changes – adaptations that may (at least in the first instance) be entirely appropriate.

The carotid, among the large arteries, has been extensively studied with regard to cardiovascular disease and the impact of hypertension. Two-dimensional ultrasound imaging can accurately measure the thickness of the arterial wall and identify local areas of plaque formation. Carotid wall thickness (specifically that of the intima media layer) increases with age and with hypertension.

In addition, most of the other recognized cardiovascular risk factors – e.g smoking, hypercholesterolaemia, diabetes, raised fibrinogen – are also associated with increased carotid wall thickness.

Increased carotid wall thickness detected by ultrasound probably represents a pre-plaque stage in the development of atherosclerosis. Subjects with greater carotid wall thickness have been shown to have a significantly increased risk of cardiovascular events. Consequently, ultrasound measurement of the carotid artery may become a clinically useful assessment of hypertension associated vascular risk.

The evidence that hypertensive structural changes occur at the level of the resistance vasculature (the smaller arteries) comes from studies of minimum forearm vascular resistance (FVR) achieved under conditions of maximum vasodilatation. The data in general show a greater 'minimum FVR' in hypertensive than in normotensive subjects. This is consistent with some fixed structural defect in the walls of small resistance arteries that restricts their calibre (Fig. 4.3). Morphological studies in animals and in humans have shown an increase in the ratio of wall thickness to lumen diameter in small arteries [12]. This structural change may be brought about by an increase in the mass of muscle present in the wall (hypertrophy), or an increase in the number of smooth muscle cells in the vessel wall (hyperplasia), or a rearrangement of the same muscle mass around a smaller lumen (remodelling). Histological studies of human vasculature in essential hypertension support the view that either hypertrophy or remodelling underlies the increase in wall-to-lumen ratio [13]. Folkow proposed that this structural change with a restricted lumen is the mechanism that maintains the elevated BP and is responsible for the amplified responses to vasoactive agents seen in hypertension (see Fig. 4.4).

Hypertension is also associated with a reduced number of small vessels in the microcirculation. This microvascular rarefaction has been observed in the retinal vascular bed, conjunctiva, mesentery, nailfold and skeletal muscle.

It remains unclear whether some or all of these 'hypertensive structural changes' in the smaller resistance circulation are cause or consequence – whether chicken or egg? Some of the features have been described in young, normotensive individuals with a family history of hypertension suggesting a causative role.

The retina offers a window for direct inspection of the small vessels. It is evident that detection of retinal vascular change in relation to hypertension offers important clues to disease progression. The retinal consequences of hypertension are dramatic (Fig.5.8), with several separate processes that may result in blindness. Severe retinal disease with accelerated or malignant hypertension is now relatively rare compared with the 1960s, because of the higher rates of screening and intervention that now prevail in most western countries; however, it remains true that advanced retinopathy and malignant hypertension are more common among hypertensive smokers. Equally, hypertension dramatically worsens retinopathy in diabetes.

Consequences of treatment

Recognition of the increased cardiovascular risk associated with hypertensive structural changes intuitively implies that regression of structural changes is a worthwhile goal in the treatment of hypertension. This is probably the case, and some prospective data support the contention. Long-term follow-up in the Framingham heart study showed that regression of electrocardiographic features of LVH confers an improvement in the risk for cardiovascular disease [14].

At all levels of hypertensive structural change – resistance vasculature, cardiac, large arteries – treatment studies demonstrate the efficacy of various therapies in achieving structural regression. The key question that remains in each case is whether the regression is proportional to the BP reduction *per se*, or is dependent on the type of treatment. In other words: 'Is there a drug-specific effect?'

Before considering this particular therapeutic question it is important to note that several of the non-pharmacological approaches to hypertension treatment – weight reduction, increased physical activity,

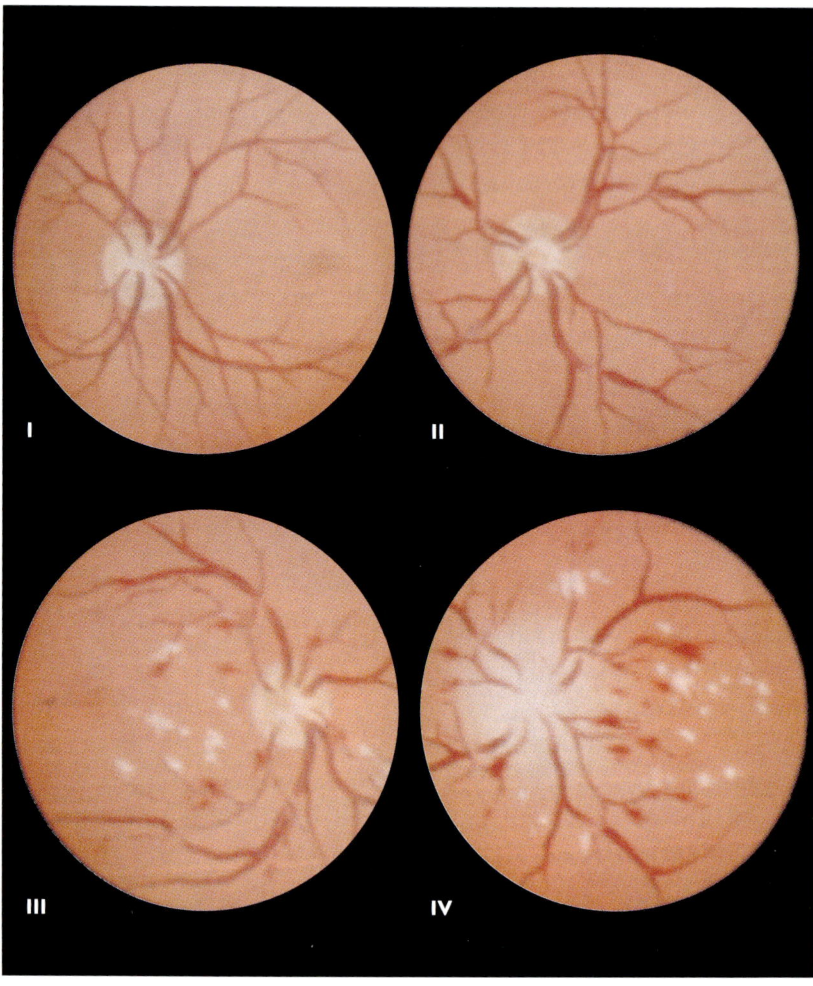

I Grade I (Keith, Wagener and Barker): Mild narrowing of the retinal arteries relative to the veins

II Grade II: Moderate sclerosis with increased light reflex and compression of veins at crossing

III Grade III: Oedema, exudates and haemorrhages; sclerotic ('silver-wire') arteries

IV Grade IV. Papilloedema, extensive haemorrhages and exudates

Figure 5.8. Gradation of retinal images through mild-to-severe retinopathy.

salt restriction – are very powerful effectors of structural regression and functional improvement. LV mass reduces with all these interventions, forearm resistance diminishes with exercise and salt restriction, and carotid wall compliance improves with exercise and salt reduction.

The structural component of FVR improves following various drug treatments, although β-blockers may be less effective in this context than other therapies. The evidence implies reversal of changes in the resistance vasculature: either reversal of remodelling and/or hypertrophy, or opening of functionally rarefied vessels or angiogenesis. Examination of small arteries from treated hypertensives has shown that effective antihypertensive treatment causes a partial improvement in the wall conformation [15].

Few treatment studies have assessed the regression of structural changes in large arteries, but these have shown a reduction in carotid wall thickness with effective BP reduction [16]. Data that compare different therapies are awaited. Regression of large artery structural changes has not yet been demonstrated to confer any benefit in terms of risk reduction. However, pathological changes in the arteries are conceptually closer to the thrombotic and haemorrhagic events of stroke and myocardial infarction than is LVH, and it is tempting to speculate that the left ventricular changes, which have hitherto been accorded such importance, merely serve as a marker for the more important arterial changes.

The clinical clustering of hypertension, dyslipidaemia, glucose intolerance and obesity (as detailed in the insulin-resistance syndrome) invites a multifaceted approach to cardiovascular disease prevention. The awareness that these risk factors, together with smoking, have supplementary adverse effects, particularly on vascular structure, reinforces the rationale for combined therapeutic approaches that include lifestyle measures and specific medications. There are strong theoretical reasons to suppose that the adverse haemodynamics and structural changes associated with hypertension synergize with elevated blood lipids, particularly low-density lipoprotein cholesterol, to result in the characteristically focal deposition of lipid particles in the arterial wall that leads to plaque formation. On these grounds a combination of lipid-lowering therapy with drugs that correct these structural and haemodynamic abnormalities should offer a powerful approach to inhibit atherogenesis. The precise structural and haemodynamic factors critical to this process and the best drugs to correct these abnormalities are clearly topics of considerable interest, but as yet remain largely unresolved. Developments in cardiovascular imaging will make it possible to address these issues in the near future.

Chapter Summary

- Increasing levels of either systolic or diastolic BP increase the risk of death.
- Systolic BP is a better predictor of subsequent cardiovascular disease than is diastolic pressure and pulse pressure is better than either systolic or diastolic in the elderly.
- The macrovascular complications of hypertension result from atherosclerotic, thrombotic and haemorrhagic vascular disease.
- The vast majority of excess deaths are due to CHD, stroke, heart failure and renal failure.
- Risk factors interact differentially with raised BP to produce stroke and CHD.
- Heart failure is now increasing because of the change in demography of the population and the success of other preventive interventions.
- LVH is an independent risk factor for CHD death.
- Coexistent diabetes leads to more complications and hypertension leads to a complex pattern of structural changes in the cardiovascular system.
- Advanced retinopathy and malignant hypertension are more common in hypertensive smokers.
- Regression of vascular structural change is a worthwhile goal.
- Clinical clustering of hypertension, dyslipidaemia, glucose intolerance and obesity suggest the need for a multifaceted approach to cardiovascular disease prevention.

References

1. Rutan GH, Kuller LH, Neaton JD, *et al.* Mortality associated with diastolic hypertension and isolated systolic hypertension among men screened for the Multiple Risk Factor Intervention Trial. *Circulation* 1998; **77**: 504–14.
2. Joint National Committee on Detection, Evaluation and Treatment of High Blood Pressure. The sixth report of the Joint National Committee on Prevention, Detection, Evaluation, and Treatment of High Blood Pressure (JNC VI). *Arch Intern Med* 1997; **157**: 2413–46.
3. Poulter NR, Sever PS, Thom S McG. *CVD: Practical Issues for Prevention*. St Albans: Caroline Black, 1996.
4. Marmot MG, Poulter NR. Primary prevention of stroke. *Lancet* 1992; **339**: 344–7.
5. Poulter NR. Is one risk factor more important than another? *Risk* 1993; **1**(2): 4–9.
6. Veterans Administration Study Group on Antihypertensive Agents. Effects of treatment on morbidity in hypertension: II. Results in patients with diastolic blood pressure averaging 90 through 114 mmHg. *J Am Med Assoc* 1970; **213**: 1143–52.
7. MacMahon S, Peto R, Cutler J, *et al.* Blood pressure, stroke, and coronary heart disease. Part I, Prolonged differences in blood pressure: prospective observational studies corrected for the regression dilution bias. *Lancet* 1990; **335**: 765–74.
8. Klahr S, Schreiner G, Ichikawa I. The progression of renal disease. *N Engl J Med* 1988; **318**: 1657–68.
9. Levy D, Larson MG, Vasan RS, *et al.* The progression from hypertension to congestive heart failure. *J Am Med Assoc* 1996; **275**: 1557–62.
10. Frohlich ED, Apstein C, Chobanian AV, *et al.* The heart in hypertension. *N Engl J Med* 1992; **327**: 998–1008.
11. Folkow B. Giraffes, rats and men – what is the importance of the 'structural factor' in normo- and hypertensive states? *Clin Exp Pharmacol Physiol* 1991; **18**: 3–11.
12. Short D. Morphology of the intestinal arterioles in chronic human hypertension. *Br Heart J* 1966; **28**: 184–92.
13. Mulvany MJ. Vascular remodelling of resistance vessels: can we define this? *Cardiovasc Res* 1999; **41**: 9–13.
14. Levy D, Salomon M, D'Agostino RB, Belanger AJ, Kannell WB. Prognostic implications of baseline electrocardiographic features and their serial changes in subjects with left ventricular hypertrophy. *Circulation* 1994; **90**: 1786–93.

15. Thybo NK, Stephens N, Cooper A, Aalkjaer C, Heagarty AM, Mulvany MJ. Effect of antihypertensive treatment on small arteries of patients with previously untreated essential hypertension. *Hypertension* 1995; **25**: 474–81.
16. Mayet J, Stanton AV, Sinclair AM. The effects of antihypertensive therapy on carotid vascular structure in men. *Cardiovascular Res* 1995; **30**: 147–52.

chapter 6

Other risk factors in hypertension

Hypertension is not a disease of the right arm, although traditional management might suggest otherwise (Fig. 6.1). The fate of patients with hypertension is modified dramatically by the coexistence of other risk factors (Fig. 6.2) and by target organ damage.

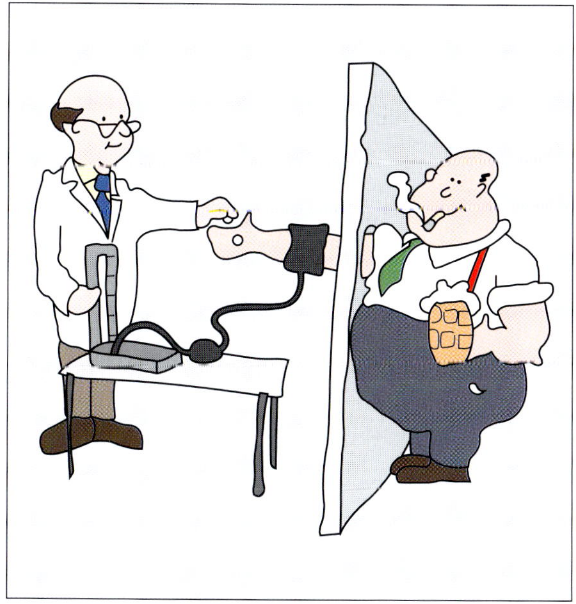

Figure 6.1. Traditional management of hypertension concentrates on the right arm alone and ignores other factors.

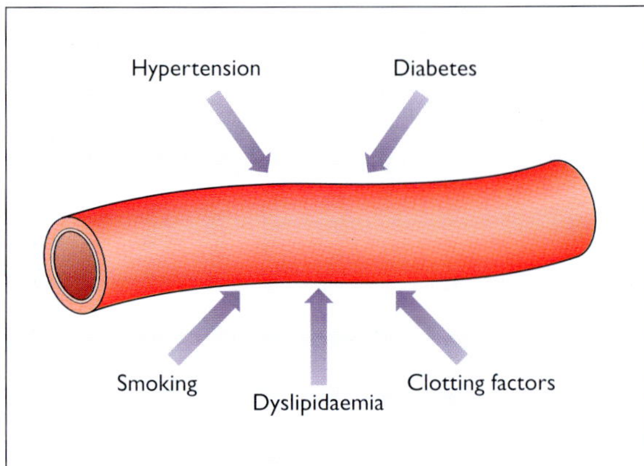

Figure 6.2. Major Risk factors for vascular damage.

COEXISTING RISK FACTORS

Hypertension is variably associated with other cardiovascular risk factors and, certainly in the UK, the majority of hypertensives have at least two other risk factors. Other risk factors tend to cluster in hypertensives more than in normotensives (Table 6.1), being commonly found in hypertensives, as shown in a recent survey of about 2000 hypertensives from 12 general practices around England (see Table 7.4) [1]. This clustering of risk factors is particularly important because, when risk factors coexist, they tend to 'interact' such that their combined adverse effect is not just greater than the sum of the individual components (additive), but is usually multiplicative or more (Fig. 6.3) [2]. For example, while the impact of elevated BP on CHD risk appears to be independent of any combination of other risk factors (Fig. 6.4 and Table 6.2) [3], it is also clear from Table 6.2 that hypertensives who smoke and are in the highest quintile of serum total cholesterol have a risk that is five times greater than hypertensives who do not smoke and have cholesterol in the lowest quintile.

The importance of the other risk factors in determining the outcome for hypertensives was also clearly demonstrated in the results of the Medical Research Council trial of hypertension (Fig. 6.5) [4]. These data show that smoking or having a total cholesterol level above

Table 6.1. Prevalence of other cardiovascular disease risk factors by BP level and sex [1]

	Total	
Risk factors	**High BP**	**Normal BP**
Men		
Alcohol >21 units/week	28	30
Cigarette smoker	20	28
Physically inactive	69	46
BMI >25 kg/m^2	77	54
Cholesterol ≥6.5 mmol/l	43	25
Women		
Alcohol >14 units/week	10	15
Cigarette smoker	18	27
Physically inactive	78	56
BMI >25 kg/m^2	66	43
Cholesterol ≥6.5 mmol/l	60	24

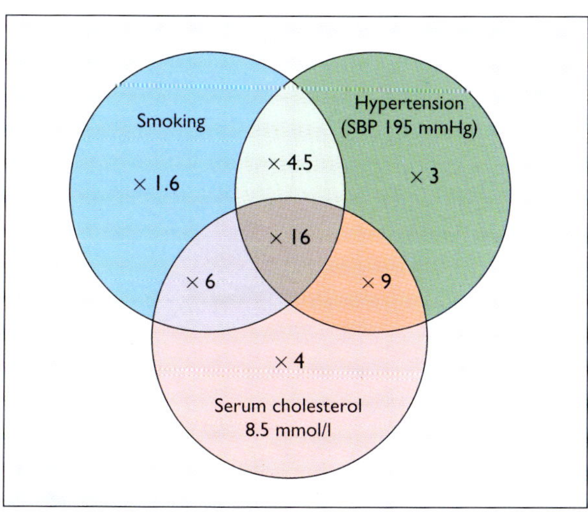

Figure 6.3. The multiplicative effect of individual components of risk.

Table 6.2. Baseline cigarette smoking, quintiles of serum cholesterol, systolic pressure and age-adjusted CHD mortality per 10 000 person-years by smoking status and quintiles of systolic BP and total cholesterol*

Serum total cholesterol (mg/dl)	Systolic BP (mmHg) <118	118–124	125–131	132–141	142+	Q5/Q1
Non-smokers						
<182	3.09	3.72	5.13	5.35	13.66	**4.4**
182–202	4.39	5.79	8.35	7.66	15.80	**3.6**
203–220	5.20	6.08	8.56	10.72	17.75	**3.4**
221–244	6.34	9.37	8.66	12.21	22.69	**3.6**
245+	12.36	12.68	16.31	20.68	33.40	**2.7**
Q5/Q1	**4.00**	**3.41**	**3.18**	**3.87**	**2.45**	–
Smokers						
<182	10.37	10.69	13.21	13.99	27.04	**2.6**
182–202	10.03	11.76	19.05	20.67	33.69	**3.4**
203–220	14.90	16.09	21.07	28.87	42.91	**2.9**
221–244	19.83	22.69	23.61	31.98	55.50	**2.8**
245+	25.24	30.50	35.26	41.47	62.11	**2.5**
Q5/Q1	**2.43**	**2.85**	**2.67**	**2.96**	**2.30**	–

*Q5 is quintile 5; Q1 is quintile 1; mean follow-up is 11.6 years; 342 815 men free of heart attack and diabetes at baseline screened for the Multiple Risk Factor Intervention Trial (MRFIT).

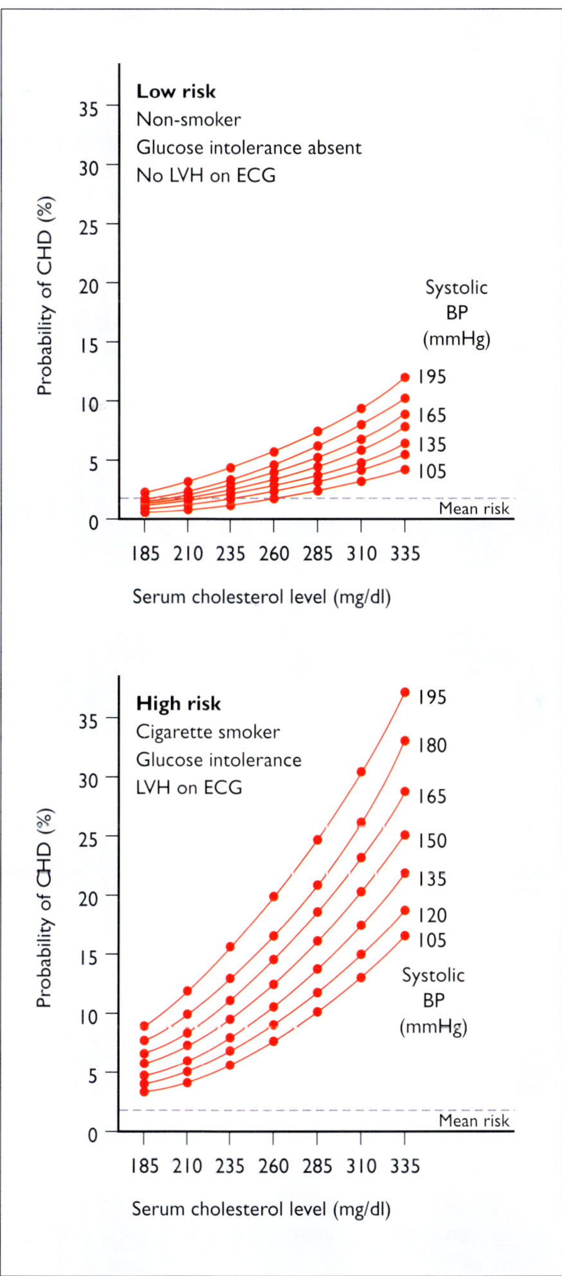

Figure 6.4. Impact of elevated BP on CHD in a low risk and a high risk population. ------ represents the mean level of population risk.

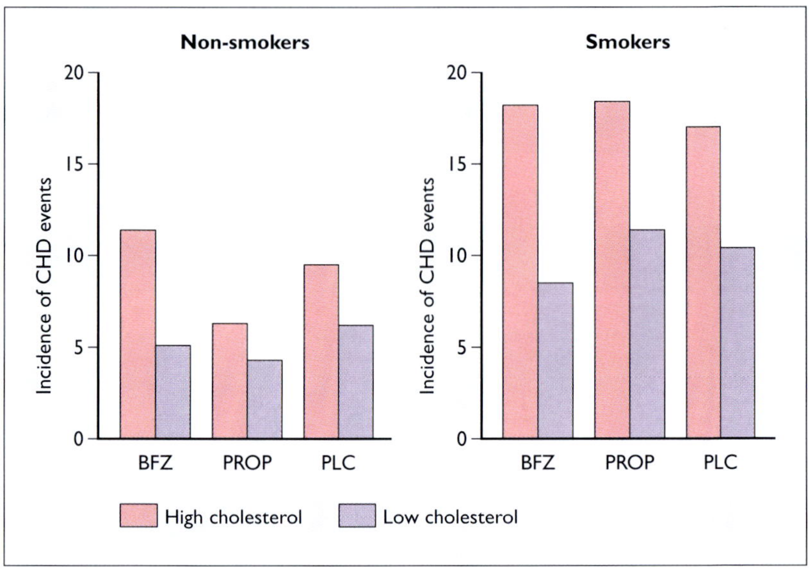

Figure 6.5. Incidence of CHD events by cholesterol and smoking. The Medical Research Council trial on hypertension. BFZ, bendrofluazide; PROP, propranolol; PLC, placebo [4].

average are stronger predictors of CHD risk than which particular anti-hypertensive agent was prescribed or even whether active BP-lowering drugs were supplied at all.

It has been proposed that hypertension forms a part of a metabolic syndrome variously referred to as 'the deadly quartet', syndrome X, Reaven's syndrome or, perhaps most suitably, the insulin-resistance syndrome [5].

Hypertension, non-insulin-dependent diabetes mellitus and obesity occur together with a greater-than-chance frequency (Fig. 6.6). Abnormalities in glucose, insulin and lipid metabolism are common to these conditions and insulin resistance is characteristic of all three. Insulin resistance is defined as impaired sensitivity to the effects of insulin on whole-body glucose uptake, but in hypertension appears to relate particularly to skeletal muscle glucose metabolism. Some of the key components of the insulin resistance syndrome are shown in Table 6.3.

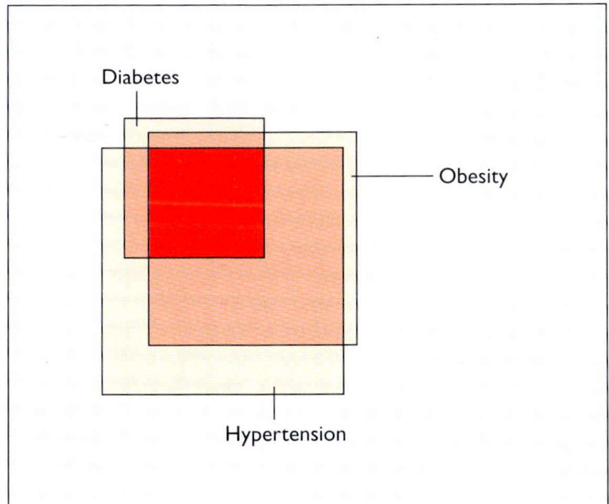

Figure 6.6. Co-occurrence of hypertension, non-insulin-dependent diabetes mellitus and obesity.

Evidence suggests that various components of the insulin-resistance syndrome are programmed in early life [6]. The excess prevalence of all the components of the insulin-resistance syndrome among South Asian communities, living in the UK and elsewhere in the world, offers the best explanation of their excessive death rate from CHD (Table 6.4) [7].

Insulin resistance is measured directly by means of concurrent glucose and insulin infusions and by quantifying the amount of

Table 6.3. Characteristics of the insulin-resistance syndrome
■ Central obesity
■ Resistance to insulin-stimulated glucose uptake
■ Glucose intolerance
■ Hyperinsulinaemia
■ Increased VLDL triglyceride
■ Decreased HDL cholesterol
■ Hypertension

Table 6.4. Risk factors for CHD in London males by ethnic group

	European (n = 1515)	South Asian (n = 1421)	African–Caribbean (n = 209)
■ Median systolic BP (mmHg)	121	126	128
■ Median diastolic BP (mmHg)	78	82	82
■ BMI (kg/m^2)	25.9	25.7	26.3
■ Total cholesterol (mmol/l)	6.11	5.98	5.87
■ Prevalence of diabetes (%)	4.8	19.6	14.6
■ Waist/hip ratio	0.94	0.98	0.94
■ HDL cholesterol (mmol/l)	1.25	1.16	1.37
■ Triglyceride (mmol/l)	1.48	1.73	1.09
■ Serum insulin (U/l)	7.2	9.8	7.1

glucose necessary to keep blood levels of glucose consistent (termed 'the insulin–glucose clamp technique'). The lower the amount of infused glucose required, the more resistant is the recipient to the hypoglycaemic effects of insulin. In more practical terms, indirect measurement of insulin resistance can be evaluated from fasting glucose and insulin levels.

It has been proposed that resistance to the insulin-mediated uptake of glucose by cells is the key to the pathophysiological links in this syndrome, and that the compensatory hyperinsulinaemia may be important in the pathogenesis of hypertension [5].

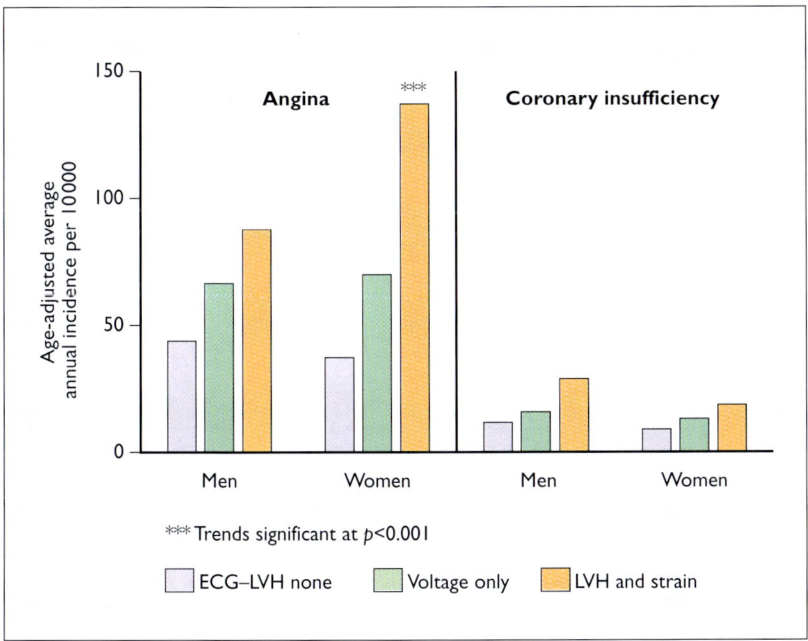

Figure 6.7. Increased levels of risk for angina and coronary insufficiency associated with the coexistence of LVH (for sudden death and myocardial infarction, see Figure 5.7).

There are several possible mechanisms whereby hyperinsulinaemia might lead to hypertension, including activation of sympathetic nerves and enhanced renal sodium and water retention. However, as yet no hypothesis is wholly convincing.

Target organ damage

As might be expected, once target organs have been damaged the risks of a major cardiovascular event associated with any given level of BP is greatly increased. For example, Figures 5.7 and 6.7 show the increased levels of risk for sudden death, myocardial infarction,

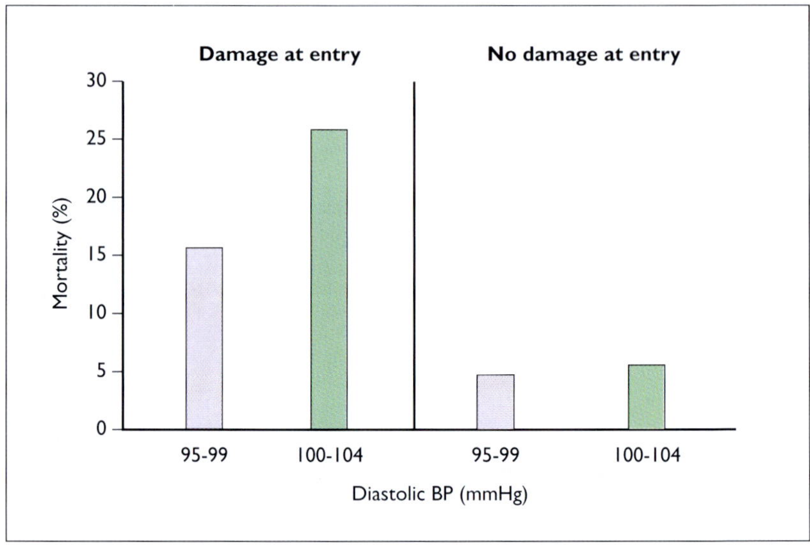

Figure 6.8. Mortality data from the Hypertension Detection and Follow-up Program by end-organ damage. 'Damage' is LVH shown by ECG or creatinine >170 mmol/l, or previous medical history of myocardial infarction, cerebrovascular accident or claudication [9].

angina and coronary insufficiency associated with the coexistence of LVH [8]. Similarly, the data shown in Figure 6.8 highlight the importance of target organ damage on the outcome of hypertensives included in the Hypertension Detection and Follow-Up Program trial [9].

Implications

Since hypertension rarely occurs in isolation from other risk factors and/or target organ damage and these problems greatly influence the outcome of patients with hypertension, it is clear that the assessment of these variables should be an integral part of the assessment of hypertensives (Chapter 7). In addition, there are implications for the targetting of both non-pharmacological management of hypertensives and the drug treatment of hypertension (Chapter 8).

CHAPTER SUMMARY

- Risk factors tend to cluster in patients with hypertension.
- Risk factors tend to interact and usually exert a multiplicative effect.
- Hypertension forms part of a metabolic syndrome variously referred to as the deadly quartet, syndrome X, Reaven's syndrome or the insulin-resistance syndrome.
- The insulin-resistance syndrome is particulary prevalent amongst South Asian communities in the UK.
- Hypertension, non-insulin-dependent diabetes mellitus and obesity occur together with a greater-than-chance frequency.
- The assessment of these variables should be an integral part of the assessment of a patient with hypertension.
- The fate of patients with hypertension is modified dramatically by the coexistence of other risk factors and by target organ damage.

References

1. Poulter NR, Zographos D, Mattin R, Sever PS, Thom S McG. Concomitant risk factors in hypertensives: a survey of risk factors for cardiovascular disease amongst hypertensives in English general practices. *Blood Pressure* 1996; **5**: 209–15.
2. Kannell W. Importance of hypertension as a major risk factor in cardiovascular disease. In: *Hypertension: Pathology and Treatment*. New York: McGraw Hill, 1997: 888–910.
3. Stamler J. Established major coronary risk factors. In: Marmot M, Elliott P, eds. *Coronary Heart Disease Epidemiology: From Aetiology to Public Health*. Oxford: Oxford University Press, 1992: 35–66.
4. Biochemical characteristics, their changes due to antihypertensive treatment, and their prognostic value. In: Miall WE, Greenberg G, on behalf of the Medical Research Coucil's Working Party on Mild to Moderate Hypertension. *Mild Hypertension – Is There Pressure to Treat?* Cambridge University Press, Cambridge, 1987: 145–52.
5. Reaven GM, Lithell H, Lansberg L. Hypertension and associated metabolic abnormalities – the role of insulin resistance and the sympathoadrenal system. *New Engl J Med* 1996; **334**: 374–81.
6. Lithell HO, McKeigue PM, Berglund L, *et al.* Relation of size at birth to non-insulin dependent diabetes and insulin concentrations in men aged 50–60 years. *Br Med J* 1996; **312**: 406–10.
7. McKeigue PM, Shah B, Marmot MG. Relation of central obesity and insulin resistance with high diabetes prevalence and cardiovascular risk in South Asians. *Lancet* 1991; **337**: 382–6.
8. Kannel WB. Prevalence and natural history of electrocardiographic left ventricular hypertrophy. *Am J Med* 1983; **75**: 4–11.
9. HDFP (Hypertension Detection and Follow-up Program) Cooperative Group. The effect of treatment on mortality in 'mild' hypertension. *New Engl J Med* 1982; **307**: 976–80.

chapter 7

Assessment of a new patient

The hypertensive patient is usually detected during the course of a routine medical examination, an employment or insurance check, or at opportunistic screening (Table 7.1). It should be considered a disaster when the diagnosis is made as a result of a vascular complication of hypertension, such as heart attack or stroke. Hypertension is one of the most common medical conditions that presents in middle-aged individuals in western society, and hence BP measurement and the search for other treatable risk factors for vascular disease is perhaps the most important preventative check that can be made in clinical practice and should be routine for all patients.

Clinical history

In the absence of vascular complications, patients with hypertension are usually symptomless and the clinical history taking and examination should be directed at finding evidence of the possible signs of target organ damage or coexistent risk factors.

A common misconception has been that hypertensive patients complain of headaches, epistaxis and lethargy; however, although occasionally headache may occur, often even severely hypertensive patients have no symptoms until they present with complications, or unless the rare situation of malignant phase hypertension arises.

History taking should focus on lifestyle, other factors for developing hypertension, previous events and symptoms that relate to the complications of hypertension and detect conditions that may affect the

Table 7.1. Basis for discovery of elevated BP

- Insurance and employment medicals
- Screening programmes
- Case-finding by general practitioners
- Health promotion clinics
- Routine measurement:
  - contraceptive pill and HRT
  - elderly
  - pregnancy

management of the patient's BP or choice of drugs (Tables 7.2 and 7.3). In the UK there is a north/south divide with a greater prevalence of risk factors in the north than in the south (Table 7.4) [1]. Note should be made as to whether or not BP has been measured in the past during an unrelated illness or when visiting the practice for other reasons, such as life insurance, pregnancy or when using the contraceptive pill.

Once the diagnosis of hypertension has been confirmed, consider the following:

- What is the level of BP?
- Are there any contributory factors (e.g. obesity, salt intake, excess alcohol intake)?
- Has the BP caused any target organ damage?
- What are the other associated cardiovascular risk factors?
- Is there any underlying cause for the increase in BP?
- Are there any contraindications to specific drugs, for example asthma (β-blockers), gout (thiazides)?

Secondary hypertension is unusual, but a focused clinical examination should aim to identify secondary causes of hypertension and complications. Coarctation of the aorta rarely gives symptoms, but may present with claudication. The diagnosis is made on clinical grounds. Renovascular disease, renal disease, phaeochromocytoma and primary

Table 7.2. History taking

- Personal history
- Age
- Sex
- Smoking and dietary habits (e.g. salt, fresh fruit and vegetable intake)
- Alcohol consumption
- Concomitant medication
- Physical activity
- Recreational drug usage
- Past and current history of coronary heart disease or cerebrovascular disease
- Diabetes
- Oral contraceptive use (and HRT)
- Respiratory illness (especially asthma or chronic obstructive airways disease)
- Family history

Table 7.3. Decision points in evaluating the hypertensive patient

Does the patient

- Have sustained hypertension?
- Take relevant drugs?
- Have hypertensive disease (effects on target organs)?
- Have other risk factors for cardiovascular disease?
- Need lifestyle modification?
- Need antihypertensive drugs?
  Is therapy urgent?
  Which drug or drugs?
- Need the minimum work-up or a more extensive search for a secondary cause or causes?
- Need a more detailed cardiovascular risk assessment?

Table 7.4. Prevalence (%) of cardiovascular disease risk factors in the UK (adapted with permission from [1])

	All (%)	North (%)	South (%)
■ Alcohol >21 units/week (males)	23.9	29.3	19.8*
■ Alcohol > 14 units/wk (females)	7.7	7.9	7.4
■ Current smoker	20.3	22.7	18.1**
■ Past smoker	43.7	40.6	46.6**
■ No exercise	70.9	75.4	67.0**
■ Total cholesterol >5.2 mmol/l	86.5	87.5	85.7
■ HDL cholesterol <0.9 mmol/l	10.3	10.6	10.0
■ History of diabetes	5.5	4.3	6.7*
■ BMI >30 kg/m^2	28.3	29.5	27.2

North versus south: *$p < 0.01$; **$p < 0.05$

aldosteronism should be excluded in the presence of unusual symptoms, early age of onset or if there are abnormalities on routine screening of renal function and electrolytes (Figs 7.1, 7.2).

A secondary cause is so unlikely that physicians often develop a negative approach. For those individuals in whom a remediable cause is found the benefits are significant. In any one individual, of course, the rarest of causes is possible and it is helpful to have some knowledge of the relative chances of particular conditions that occur in order to target appropriate history taking and investigations (Fig. 7.1).

Past history

Past history may well give clues as to the presence of secondary causes of hypertension; particularly seek for past renal disease or evidence of previous vascular complications of raised BP. In women a detailed

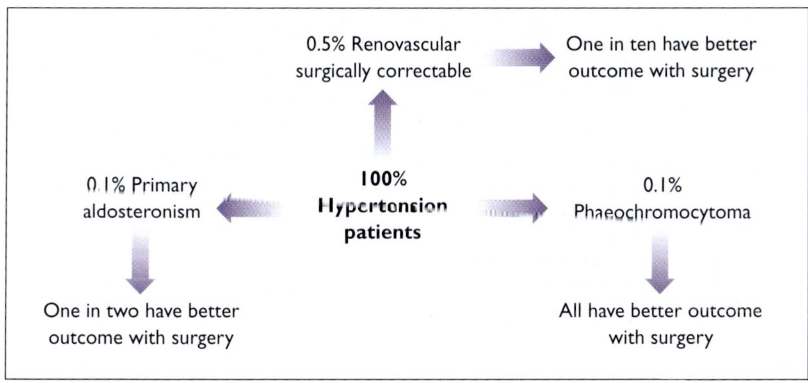

Figure 7.1. Prevalence of secondary hypertension.

obstetric history is necessary with regard to previous pre-eclampsia pregnancy related hypertension or hypertension caused by the OC pill.

Family history

Family history of hypertension is common (Fig. 7.3), but other useful indicators are a history of premature death, heart attack, or stroke. Adult polycystic renal disease is inherited as a Mendelian dominant condition. A family history of diabetes alerts the physician that the patient may be diabetic. A family history of hyperlipidaemia is relevant and patients with hypertension should be advised to tell their relatives to have their BP measured.

Social history

The risk of complications depends to some extent upon genetic susceptibility to cardiovascular disease, but environmental factors such as diet, alcohol, physical activity and smoking are important. Hypertension is more common in people of lower socioeconomic groups, but is not associated with any particular occupational groups and is not necessarily associated with stressful jobs. A high alcohol

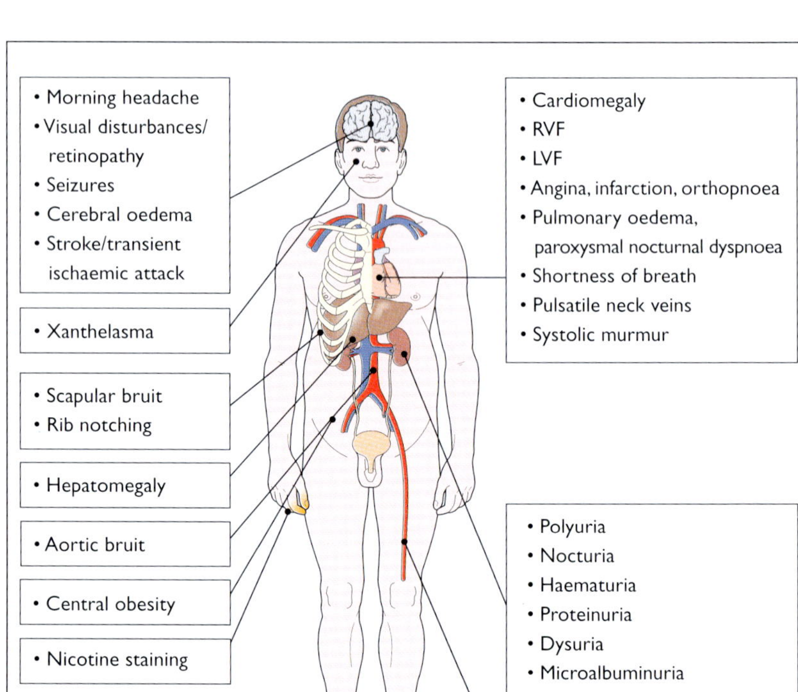

Figure 7.2. Symptoms and signs of hypertension.

intake is closely related to high BP, an effect independent of age, sex, personality, cigarette smoking or salt consumption. A healthy diet should be encouraged; in particular patients should be asked if they consume large quantities of salt by adding it to their food or by eating large amounts of processed foods. Cigarette smoking is an independent cardiovascular risk factor, but interacts very strongly with other important risk factors such as hypercholesterolaemia and hypertension (see Chapter 6).

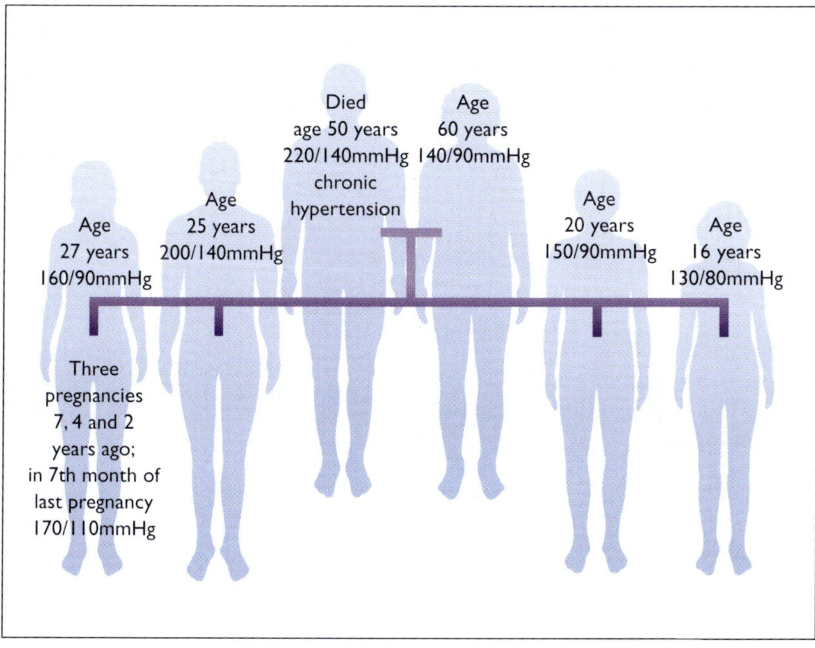

Figure 7.3. The impact of inheritable and environmental factors on hypertension. A typical family tree with hypertension in the father (who died of a stroke), showing the variable occurrence of a raised BP in the children, which is partly dependent upon age but is also exposed by pregnancy.

Drug history

It is important to discover whether or not the patient has been treated previously for hypertension, and whether or not the patient is currently taking any antihypertensive medication. In addition to this, any previous intolerance to any drugs for hypertension must be established. Some drugs, notably the oral contraceptive and steroids, can cause hypertension, and there may be interactions with psychotropic and nonsteroidal anti-inflammatory drugs (Table 7.5). Accurate documentation of any concomitant medication is important.

Table 7.5. Drugs that affect BP

- **Drugs that cause sodium retention**
  Oral corticosteroids
  Adrenocorticotrophic hormone
  Carbenoxolone
  Nonsteroidal anti-inflammatory drugs
- **Drugs that cause increased sympathomimetic activity**
  Ephedrine, cocaine and amphetamines
  Cold cures
  Monoaminoxidase inhibitors
- **Direct vasoconstrictors**
  Ergot alkaloids
- **Combined oral contraceptives**
- **Interactions with antihypertensive drugs**
  Nonsteroidal anti-inflammatory drugs
  Tricyclic antidepressants

Physical examination

Physical examination should include a search for the causes and effects of hypertension and for evidence of other cardiovascular risk factors and diseases that may affect the choice of management (Fig. 7.2). Weight should be measured – this provides a baseline for future measurements. General examination incorporates identifying conditions such as Cushing's syndrome, acromegaly, coarctation, renal artery stenosis and xanthelasmata which are associated with hyperlipidaemia. Nicotine staining of the fingers is an important physical sign.

Examination of the cardiovascular system

The BP should be measured in a standardized fashion on several occasions and, in certain circumstances, ambulatory monitoring should be considered (see Chapter 3). The pulse may be of large volume and there may be a tachycardia if the patient is anxious. There may be some thickening of the vessel wall, caused by arteriosclerosis. All the peripheral pulses should be checked and the carotid and femoral pulses auscultated for bruits. The femoral pulses are checked for volume and delay, which suggests coarctation of the aorta. The cardiac apex is palpated and the presence or absence of LVH noted. In the presence of raised BP the aortic component of the second heart sound is loud, and if there is a failing left ventricle, a third heart sound or gallop rhythm may be heard.

Careful attention should be paid to the presence or absence of cardiac murmurs, since hypertension can coexist with cardiac valve disease. Ejection systolic murmurs are common in hypertension and aortic valve disease should be considered, particularly if a thrill is palpable, if the murmur is of a high grade or if the aortic component of the second heart sound is quiet, which suggests aortic stenosis.

Coarctation of the aorta may be associated with a loud systolic murmur over the left precordium with radiation into the left scapular region, where pulsation may be palpable.

Auscultation of the chest may reveal the presence of basal crepitations, suggesting left ventricular failure; the presence or absence of obstructive airways disease should be determined.

The abdomen is examined with particular attention to the size of the liver and kidneys and renal bruits, although an insensitive sign, may suggest renal artery stenosis.

The central nervous system is examined to detect neurological defect caused by cerebrovascular disease and the examination of the optic fundi should be an integral part of the assessment of every hypertensive patient. The eye is an important site for damage caused by hypertension and is unique because blood vessels can be visualized directly. The use of a short-acting mydriatic greatly facilitates the technique. Ophthalmoscopy rapidly identifies those patients with malignant hypertension and is particularly helpful in the elderly, in whom it can reveal important causes of visual loss caused by hypertension (Table 7.6, Figs 7.4–7.7; see also Chapter 5).

Table 7.6. Features seen on fundoscopy in hypertensive patients

Feature	Interpretation
Increased arterial tortuosity	This may be age related
Silver wiring	This suggests arterial wall thickening and is common in older patients
Arteriovenous nipping	Caused by pressure on the retinal veins by thickening retinal arteries
Retinal flame-shaped haemorrhages	Occur in severe hypertension
Cotton-wool spots	Are retinal infarcts that cause exudation
Hard, shiny exudates	These are lipid-laden
Early signs of disc oedema	Caused by overfilling of the veins, loss of the venous pulsation, hyperaemia of the nerve head and blurring both of the disc margin and details of the physiological cup.

Any patient who has persistent high BP should have some further investigations, particularly the young, and in those patients suspected to have renal impairment. If control is difficult secondary causes must be excluded.

Investigation of hypertensive patients

The British Hypertension Society (BHS) [2] recommends that routine investigation should be limited to:

- Urine strip test for blood and protein
- Serum creatinine and electrolytes
- Blood glucose
- Serum total:HDL cholesterol
- ECG

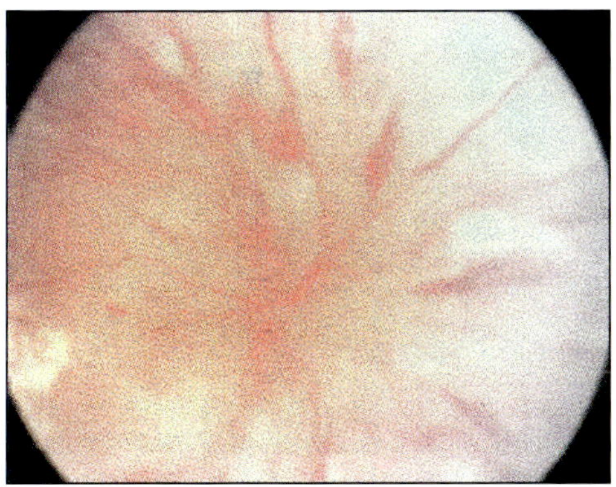

Figure 7.4. Malignant hypertension. Gross papilloedema is seen with the vessels on the disc obscured. Flame haemorrhages, cotton-wool exudates and retinal oedema occur at all areas.

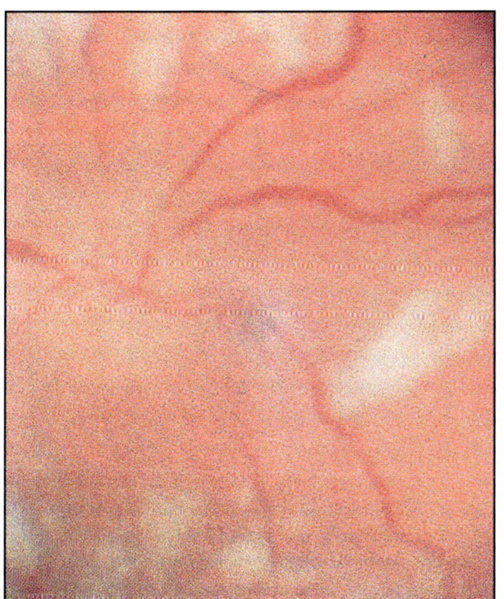

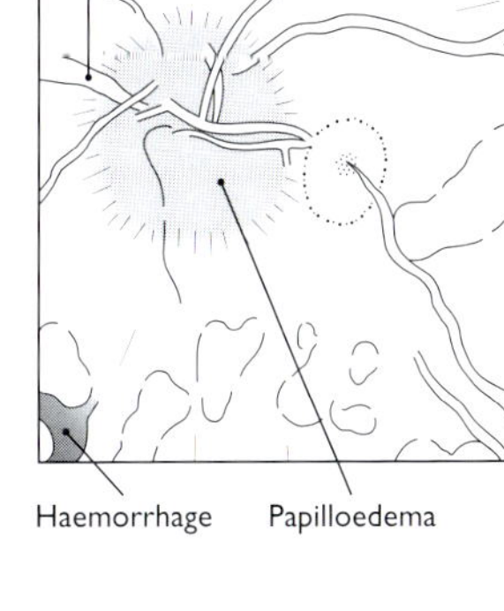

Figure 7.5. Malignant hypertension. Papilloedema and numerous cotton-wool exudates are seen at all areas with a solitary haemorrhage.

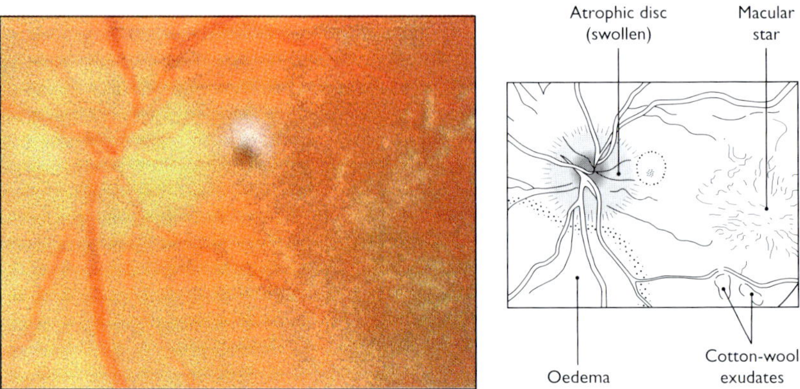

Figure 7.6. Malignant hypertension. Papilloedema developing into a white atrophic appearance of the disc. A striking macular star figure with a red, rather haemorrhagic appearance at the centre, which is the macula. Retinal oedema is present, particularly below the disc. The arteries are very narrow.

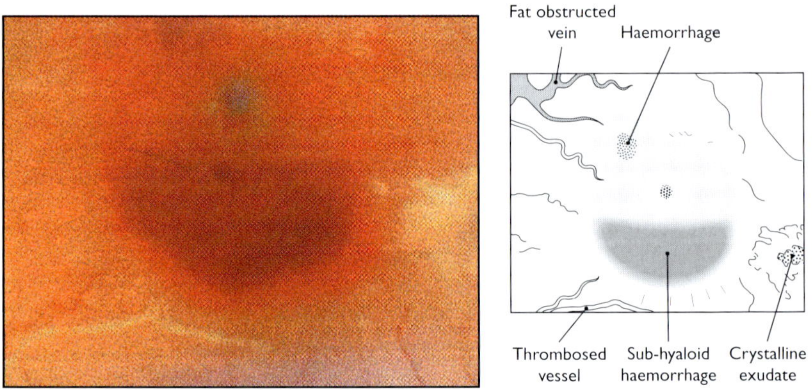

Figure 7.7. A large subhyaloid haemorrhage with a typical straight upper and curved lower margin, like a cup. There are clear-cut, rather crystalline exudates on the outer side, a type often seen in diabetes (which this patient had). Below the haemorrhage is a white thrombosed vessel.

However, the clinical history and may suggest the need for further investigation (see Chapter 10), for example:

- Full blood count and γGTP if there is a suspicion of alcohol excess
- Uric acid if there is a history of gout or renal disease
- Urine for catecholamines if the history suggests phaeochromocytoma
- Ultrasound of kidneys or intravenous pyelography if renal disease is suspected.

Note that chest radiography, urine microscopy and culture and echocardiography are not required routinely. Echo is valuable to confirm or refute the presence of LVH when the ECG shows a 'high' left ventricular voltage without T-wave abnormalities, as is often the case in young patients. When the results and clinical evaluation of these simple investigations suggest a need for further investigations, it is usually best to refer for specialist advice, because some of the additional investigations needed are often difficult to arrange from general practice[2].

The interpretation of common abnormalities on blood tests in newly diagnosed hypertensive patients is given in Table 7.7.

Examination of the urine may show blood or protein. If haematuria is found, red cells are sought in a midstream specimen. It may be found in patients with malignant hypertension and glomerular diseases, but bladder neoplasia must be excluded. Proteinuria is common, especially in malignant hypertension and in those patients with underlying renal disease. An ECG should be performed on all newly diagnosed hypertensive patients and may provide evidence of LVH or strain. It may also show undetected arythmias and evidence of previous myocardial infarction or ischaemia and it is very useful as a record if ischaemia develops subsequently. When there is evidence of LVH the risk associated with a given BP is much increased and echocardiography is useful to confirm the degree of hypertrophy and to monitor the response to treatment.

Table 7.7. Interpretation of blood tests in newly diagnosed hypertensive patients

Test	Interpretation
Sodium	High (142–150 mmol/l) in patients with primary aldosteronism May be low, in heavy drinkers and in those taking diuretics
Potassium	Low in primary and secondary aldosteronism; however, the most common cause of hypokalaemia is diuretic treatment
Bicarbonate	Metabolic alkalosis with an increased plasma bicarbonate can result from primary aldosteronism or diuretic treatment
Urea and creatinine	Gives a crude guide to renal function; even small increases of creatinine concentration should suggest the need for further investigations, particularly for an underlying renal cause
Uric acid	May be elevated in about 40% of hypertensive patients, especially in renal disease and with heavy drinking
Total and HDL cholesterol (non-fasting sample will suffice)	Abnormalities should be treated aggressively in all hypertensive patients
Blood glucose	Diabetes is more common in the hypertensive population; the presence of diabetes requires extra attention to good BP control
Full blood count	An increase in MCV may indicate excessive alcohol consumption or polycythaemia may suggest heavy smoking

Assessment in Context

In patients with hypertension it is appropriate to assess the absolute risk of CHD – that is the probability of developing nonfatal myocardial infarction or fatal CHD over a defined time period given a particular combination of risk factors – and to intervene appropriately depending on the degree to which they are at risk. Taking account of all the major cardiovascular risk factors avoids undue emphasis being placed on an individual risk factor at the expense of overall or absolute risk.

As a minimum, apparently healthy individuals with a 30% or higher CHD risk over 10 years should also be identified and treated appropriately and effectively. As the scientific evidence clearly justifies risk-factor intervention in healthy individuals with a CHD risk lower than 30%, it is entirely appropriate as the next step to seek out and treat those with a lower risk. One method would be to take the opportunity to screen and identify those individuals with a 15% or more CHD risk over 10 years, as long as those at the high levels of risk have already received effective preventive care.

The computer program 'Cardiac risk assessor' developed for these recommendations is the preferred method of calculating absolute 10-year CHD risk for an individual, and is based on the Framingham Function. It can also be used to calculate cardiovascular risk (including stroke over the same period). However, this is a computer method and may not be convenient in all clinical settings and therefore the coronary risk chart (see Fig. 8.8) can also be used to identify those healthy individuals at highest CHD risk (30% or higher – red band), those at the next level of CHD risk (15% or higher – orange band), and finally those whose CHD risk is less than 15% (green band) [3].

Table 7.8. Management of hypertension

- Measure BP correctly
- Observe for a variable period according to severity
- Evaluate overall risk profile
- Treat all hypertensives with additional non-pharmacological measures
- Recognize the efficacy limitations of individual hypertensive drugs
- Consider the impact of side effects on quality of life
- Recognize that poor compliance is common
- Review regularly to ensure BP control is maintained and other risk factors are improved
- Adopt a multidisciplinary approach that involves the practice nurse

MANAGING HYPERTENSION

The approach required to manage hypertension is given in Table 7.8 At present, available treatment options for hypertension include:

- Diuretics
- β-blockers
- ACE inhibitors
- Calcium antagonists
- α_1 adrenoceptor blockers
- Angiotensin II antagonists
- Other agents, such as moxonidine

Chapter Summary

- Hypertension is one of the most common medical conditions to present in middle-aged individuals in western society.
- Raised BP is usually asymptomatic and may remain silent for many years.
- Every opportunity should be taken to incorporate BP measurements into a patient's visits to the PHCT, irrespective of the cause of the visit.
- Establish any contributory factors.
- Establish any target organ damage caused by the BP.
- Establish other associated cardiovascular risk factors.
- Underlying causes for the increase in BP must be sought.
- Seek contraindications to specific drugs.
- Routine investigations should be limited to urine strip test for blood and protein, serum creatinine and electrolytes, blood glucose, serum total:HDL cholesterol and ECG.
- The decision to undertake additional investigations or refer to secondary care depends on the clinical evaluation, the results of the initial investigations, the level of BP and also the presence of other risk factors.
- Evaluate the overall risk profile.
- Adopt a multidisciplinary approach that involves the practice nurse.

References

1. Poulter NR, Zographos D, Mattin R, Sever PS, Thom SMcG. Concomitant risk factors in hypertensives: a survey of risk factors for cardiovascular disease among hypertensives in English general practices. *Blood Pressure* 1996: **5**; 209–15.
2. Ramsay LE, Johnston GD, MacGregor GA, *et al*. Guidelines for management of hypertension: report of the Third Working Party of the British Hypertension Society 1999. *J Hum Hypertens* 1999; **13**: 569–92.
3. Wood D, Durrington P, McInnes G, Poulter N, Rees A, Wray R on behalf of the British Cardiac Society, British Hyperlipidaemia Association, British Hypertension Society, British Diabetic Association. Joint British recommendations on prevention of coronary heart disease in clinical practice. *Heart* 1998; **80(Suppl. 2)**:S1–S29.

Further reading

MacGregor GA, Kaplan NM. *Fast Facts – Hypertension*. Abingdon: Health Press, 1998.

O'Brien ET, Beevers DG, Marsall HJ. *ABC of Hypertension*. London: BMJ Publishing, 1995.

Swales JD. *Textbook of Hypertension*. Oxford: Blackwell Science, 1994.

chapter 8

Prevention and management of hypertension

There are essentially two basic strategies – high risk and population based – that can be employed to prevent diseases that result from high BP.

The majority of the preventive effort is currently directed towards the high-risk strategy, that is screening large numbers of people in an attempt to identify those with elevated BP and, having confirmed BP elevation, initiating treatment(s). To be fully successful, this strategy depends on the identification and completely effective treatment of all hypertensives. Such a strategy has the effect shown in Figure 8.1, and

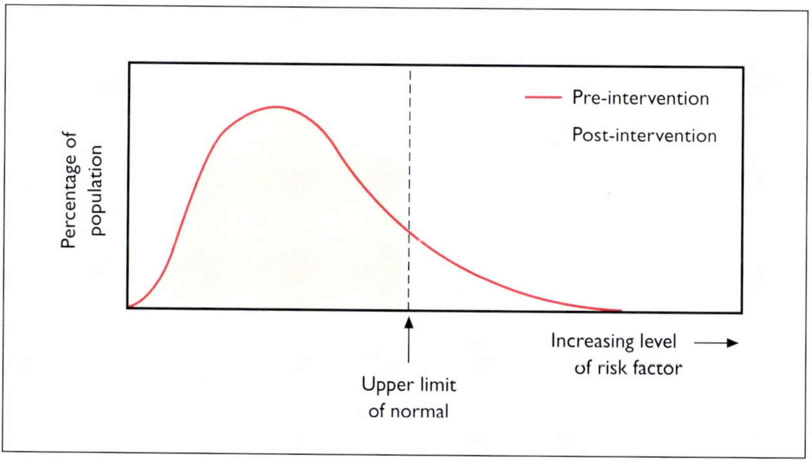

Figure 8.1. Effect of successful identification and treatment of all hypertensives.

Table 8.1. High-risk strategy

For	Against
■ Intervention apparently appropriate ■ Subject and doctor motivated ■ Ratio of 'costs' (e.g. side effects) to benefits favourable ■ Cost effective	■ Costs: financial and other (e.g. labelling people as patients) ■ Difficulties of screening ■ Palliative rather than radical approach ■ Limited potential ■ Behaviourally difficult (making changes after many years) ■ Too late in the pathological process

the advantages and disadvantages of this approach are shown in Table 8.1. The major problem from a population viewpoint is that the majority of adverse events attributable to raised BP occur below the 'hypertensive' range (see Table 5.1). Consequently, most adverse sequelae of hypertension are unaffected by a high-risk strategy.

The alternative population approach is essentially an attempt to move the distribution of BP in the whole population downwards. If successful, this approach has the effect shown in Figure 8.2. It has been estimated that a downwards shift of about 2.5 mmHg in diastolic BP from the population's mean BP would generate the same degree of benefits that accrue from the high-risk strategy as currently practised [1]. The advantages and disadvantages of this approach are shown in Table 8.2.

These two strategies should not be considered mutually exclusive. Optimal benefits, in terms of reducing hypertension-induced cardiovascular disease, are likely to be achieved by an effective integrated application of both strategies. The population strategy requires input from government, education and industry, whereas the high-risk strategy is seen to be the role of the medical and allied professions.

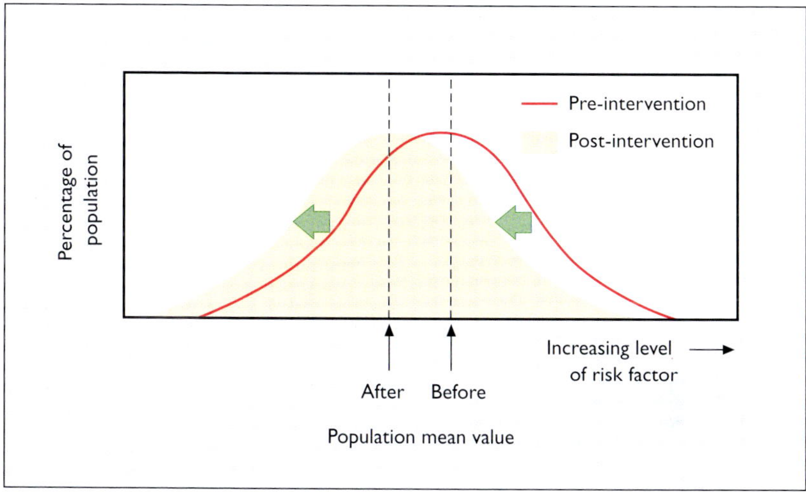

Figure 8.2. Effect of moving the distribution of BP in the whole population downwards.

Table 8.2. Population strategy

For	Against
■ Radical	■ Small individual benefit
■ Greater potential for the population as a whole	■ Limited motivation for the medical profession
■ Easy to maintain a healthy lifestyle throughout life when considered 'the norm'	■ Therapeutic ratio (i.e. benefits:costs) difficult to evaluate and may cause concern

However, acknowledgement of the potential benefits of the population strategy should have implications regarding the global application of non-pharmacological advice to lower BP.

Table 8.3. Non-pharmacological interventions

- Weight reduction to ideal body weight
- Regular physical exercise
- Limit alcohol consumption (men <21 units/week; women <14 units/week)
- Reduce dietary salt intake
- Increase fruit and vegetable intake
- Reduce total and saturated fat intakes
- Stop smoking

All the recent national and international guidelines for hypertension management are unanimous in recommending non-pharmacological treatments for all hypertensive patients, irrespective of the severity of the BP elevation [2–6]. The rationale for so doing is that each of the recommended non-pharmacological interventions shown in Table 8.3 (except smoking cessation) has been shown in various types of studies to reduce BP, over and above the BP reductions induced by drug therapy. Furthermore, in recent years, increasingly trial evidence has demonstrated the benefits of various non-pharmacological manoeuvres in terms of the prevention and treatment of hypertension. Consequently, by using non-pharmacological means, the need for drugs will be pre-empted in a proportion of patients, and in those who require drug therapy the number of drugs required will be reduced, as will the doses of whatever drugs are used.

The universal recommendation, made in all the guidelines, to stop smoking is because, although clinic BP is unlikely to fall after smoking cessation, the benefit in terms of cardiovascular risk reduction is greatly enhanced when two or more risk factors are reduced because of the multiplicative effect on risk when two risk factors coexist (see Chapter 6).

STOPPING SMOKING

The *Smoking Cessation Guidelines for Health Professionals* [7], which is also published in summary form [8], is a very useful document for physicians trying to help their patients to stop smoking. Advice to patients on how to stop smoking should recognize the powerful addictive property of nicotine and the strong association between routine daily events and smoking habits. Successful treatment regimens often include the principle of gradual nicotine withdrawal, together with simple behavioural reprogramming. Such plans are designed to break the immediate association of particular events with smoking cigarettes in a positive rather than a negative manner. The number of cigarettes and their nicotine content may gradually be reduced over a 3–4 week period, before a predetermined cut-off date after which no cigarettes are smoked.

The use of nicotine replacement therapy (with patches, gum, nasal sprays and inhalators) holds promise in assisting phased smoking withdrawal. As these replacement therapies roughly double cessation rates irrespective of adjunctive support, they should be routinely recommended to smokers. It must be recognized that most people who finally do give up smoking have tried to do so on several previous occasions, so support and encouragement for those who relapse is a logical and important approach.

A more active governmental anti-smoking policy is required. A tobacco advertising ban, although promised in a protracted way, has yet to be enforced in the UK. As long as the European Community continues to subsidize the European farming of tobacco exported to developing countries, the fight against smoking may appear to be an uphill struggle. However, health professionals should be encouraged because the most common explanation offered by ex-smokers of why they gave up is 'My doctor told me to!' Most have, in fact, given up smoking by themselves without further professional assistance.

Weight loss

The association between weight loss and a fall in BP has been clearly demonstrated in a meta-analysis of several studies [9], and weight loss may enhance the response to BP-lowering drugs. However, it has to be acknowledged that persuading patients to lose weight is not easy. It is not surprising that the medical profession are frequently ineffective and defeatist in this area, given the absence hitherto of teaching on communication skills, nutrition and dietetics in medical school curricula. The provision of more trained dieticians to support better informed medical advice may well be a cost-effective long-term measure to reduce cardiovascular disease. Furthermore, gains may be made if the food industry can be persuaded to reduce the salt content of their products, to provide clear food labelling to help consumer choice and to give price incentives to promote healthier products. The following general points may help to achieve effective weight loss:

- The adviser should be well-informed, clear, committed and show enthusiasm, while providing time, understanding, positive feedback and follow-up.
- The diet should be discussed in the context of the whole family, the cook, cooking methods and practical guidance about shopping.
- Advice should not consist of a draconian list of negatives, but rather alternative foods should be suggested that will maintain an adequate nutritional balance and avoid nagging hunger.
- Fresh fruit and vegetables are filling and usually low in calories. For this and other reasons (see sodium and potassium intake below) their consumption should be strongly encouraged.
- Weight should be lost gradually over a prolonged period. Hence the need for reinforcement, and encouragement from the counsellor.
- Reduced fat intake is a particularly effective method of reducing body weight.
- Reduce salt intake.
- The same number of calories subdivided into several small meals puts on less weight than the same number of calories consumed in one large meal, particularly if the large meal is eaten last thing at night.

The independent effect of these measures on BP levels has been controversial. However, recently the benefits of a low fat diet on BP levels were clearly demonstrated in the Dietary Approaches to Stop Hypertension (DASH) trial (Fig. 8.3) [10]. In addition to this direct effect on BP, low fat intake has the advantage of enhancing weight loss and improving lipid profiles. The latter effect has received 'bad press', but the incorrectly held belief that dieting does not affect lipids results from confusion over the answers to two questions. The first question is whether dietary measures, if adhered to, lower lipids. The answer is they do, with the reasonable expectation that total cholesterol falls by about 10% on average, given reasonable dietary manoeuvres [10]. The second problem is whether we are effective at

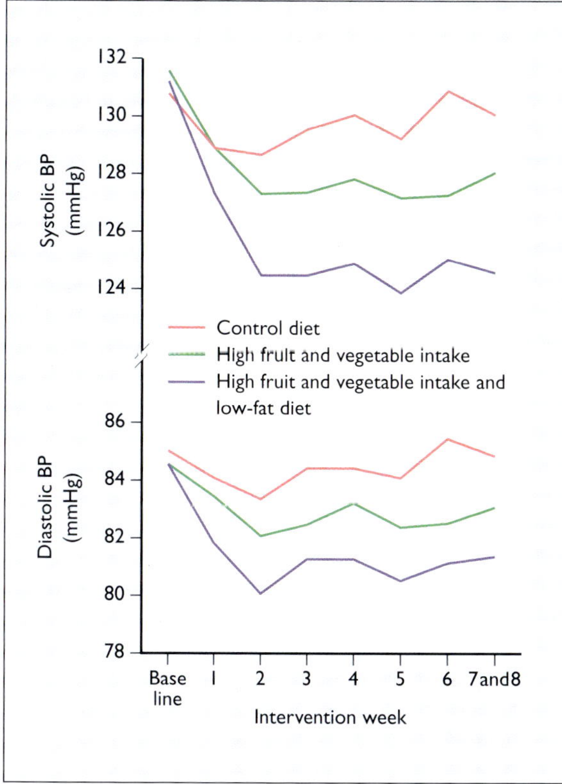

Figure 8.3. Mean systolic and diastolic BPs at baseline and during each intervention week, by diet. Adapted from Appel *et al.* [10].

persuading our patients to change their diets. The answer is we are not, which has been misinterpreted to mean that dietary intervention does not work. The effect of various lifestyle manoeuvres on lipid subfractions is shown in Table 8.4.

It is a widely held misconception that 'red meat' is the source of all saturated fat and related evils. However, there is more fat in a piece of vegetarian quiche than there is in a grilled lean steak!

ALCOHOL RESTRICTION

Alcohol, possibly by means of a direct effect on blood vessels and possibly by increasing sympathetic tone, appears to increase BP [11]. Alcohol withdrawal studies showed that, although acute withdrawal (i.e. hangover) may cause elevated BP, thereafter BP levels are reduced (Fig. 8.4). It is important to note that not only do population studies show that BP levels are generally higher on Mondays than those later in the week, but also that admission to hospital for stroke is most common at the weekend. Such observations are likely to be linked to the increased alcohol consumption that occurs at the weekend. Other data suggest that abstinence during the week with heavy consumption at the weekend is probably worse than drinking the same total amount of alcohol evenly spread throughout the week. Although the UK government in the 1990s raised the recommended upper limits for sensible drinking, the rationale for so doing was not based on scientific evidence. Certainly among hypertensives, the number of units (Fig. 8.5) should be restricted to no more than 21 (for men) or 14 (for women) units per week.

Special advice is needed for patients whose social life is built around the pub, such as:

- Change the type of beer or lager drunk to a brand that contains less alcohol (several low-alcohol beers and lagers are available on draught and in cans).
- Add soda water to wine (a spritzer); this is only helpful if the total amount of wine consumed is reduced!

Table 8.4. The effects of dietary and lifestyle variables on serum lipid profiles

Variable	LDL	HDL	Triglyceride
Dietary saturated fat	↑	↓	↑
Dietary polyunsaturated fat	↓	↓	↓
Dietary monounsaturated fat	↓	–	↓
Alcohol	?	↑	↑
Exercise	↓	↑	↓
Smoking	–	↓	↑
Excess body weight	↑	↓	↑
Fish oil	↓	–	↓
Soluble fibre	↓	–	—

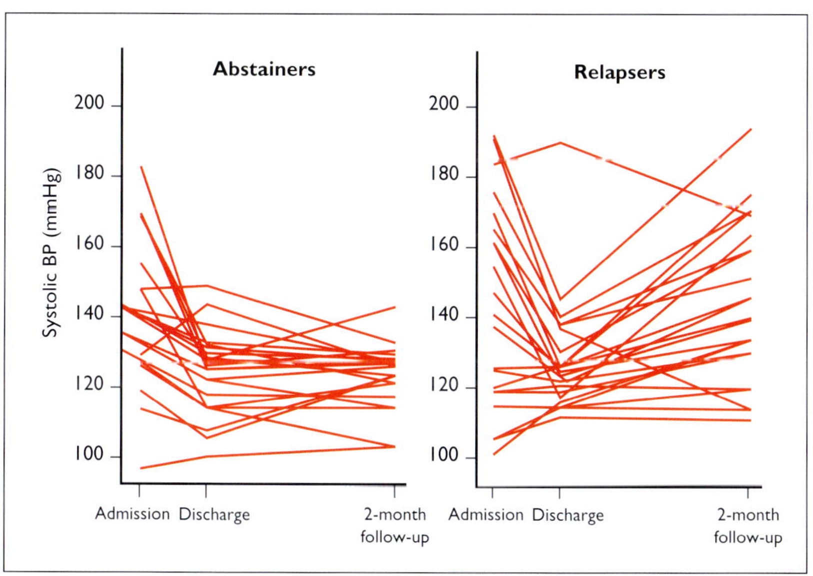

Figure 8.4. Effects of alcohol abstention and relapse.

One unit of alcohol =
Half a pint of beer
One glass of wine
One measure of spirits

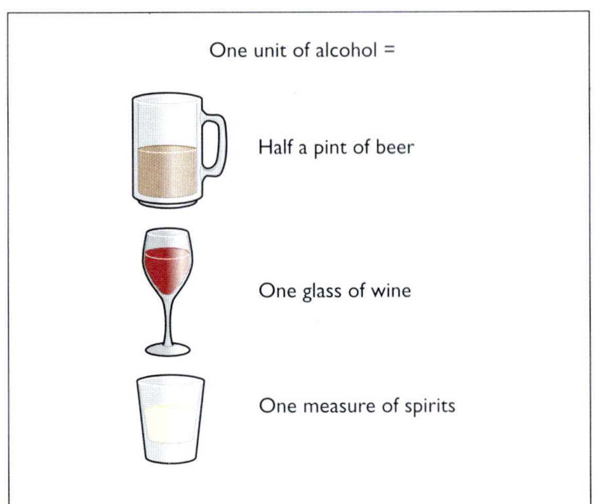

Figure 8.5. Units of alcohol.

Sodium and potassium intake

Although individual responses vary, a lower dietary salt intake reduces average BP levels, particularly in the elderly. The results of 78 trials of the effects of modification of salt intake and BP confirmed the findings of observational studies in that the association of BP with sodium intake was larger than generally appreciated and increased with age and initial BP [12]. Furthermore, all trials in which salt restriction was added to drug therapy (with the possible exception of those that studied calcium antagonists) show an additional affect of BP lowering associated with salt restriction.

The relationship between sodium and BP described in Chapter 4 indicates that a dietary reduction of 100 mmol of sodium is associated with a 6 mmHg reduction in systolic BP.

Recommending the reduction of salt in the diet requires specific advice, because it is not generally appreciated that sodium is found in remarkably high quantities in many commonly consumed foods such as bread. Patients need to be told of this and to be warned off high-salt foods (e.g. Marmite, Oxo cubes, processed and canned foods).

In view of the possible protective effects of increasing potassium in the diet, particularly against stroke, it is reasonable to recommend foods rich in potassium, particularly since these foods (fruit and vegetables) tend to have healthy profiles independent of their potassium content (n.b., patients with renal failure should avoid high potassium diets). Dried figs, mushrooms and orange juice are high in potassium content and bananas contain 1 mmol of potassium per inch!

It is estimated that a dietary increase of 100 mmol/day of potassium is associated with a 10 mmHg reduction in systolic BP and an increase of 100 mmol/day has been associated with a 40% reduction in stroke mortality amongst a large cohort of elderly people [13].

Physical exercise

Studies suggest that regular aerobic exercise induces a moderate BP lowering effect [14]. However the effects of exercise also include benefits in terms of improved lipid profiles, insulin resistance, body weight, cardiac training and general well-being (Fig. 8.6). Some data also suggest that regular exercise assists in coping with stress.

The medical profession and the general population need to be convinced of the benefits and safety of exercise, which would promote enthusiasm for physically active lifestyles. However, enthusiasm needs accessible facilities if sporting activities are to be increasingly adopted. Ideally, enthusiasm should be engendered at school.

To achieve the optimal benefit, exercise should be regular, but it does not necessarily need to be vigorous. Indeed, it is clear from data presented in a recent review of the benefits of exercise that, in what is essentially a sedentary society, minimal increases in activity are likely to induce cardiovascular benefits (Fig 8.7) [15]. Data from various studies show that brisk walking is sufficiently vigorous to induce cardiovascular training in more than two-thirds of the population. For further benefits activity should be built up gradually to a level that doubles the pulse rate. The exercise should be repeated at least three

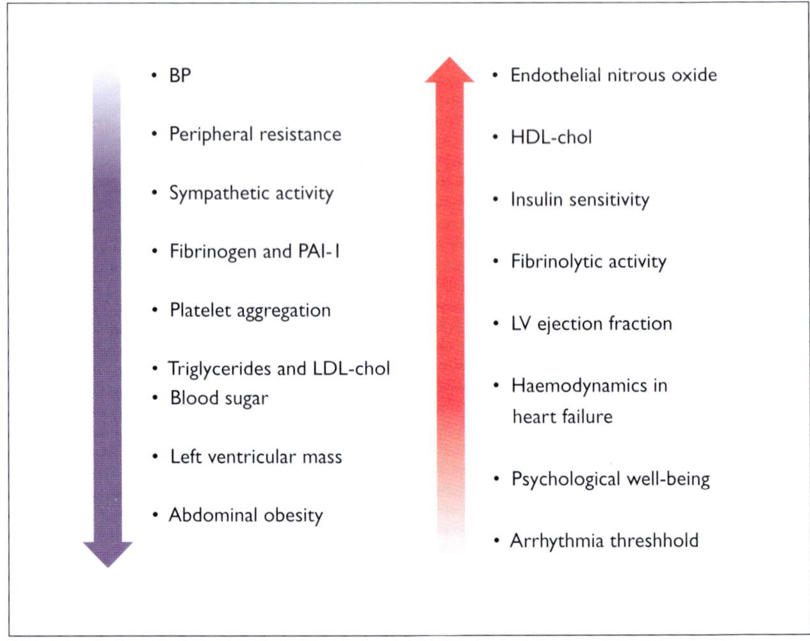

Figure 8.6. Potential mechanisms underlying the cardiovascular benefits of exercise.

times weekly for about 20 minutes each session. The style of exercise recommended is largely aerobic (e.g. walking, swimming, cycling) rather than isometric muscle work, such as weight lifting, which can cause extreme rises in BP.

Concern is frequently expressed about the risks of vigorous exercise because of the modestly increased risk of sudden death at the time of the exercise, particularly in those unaccustomed to it. However, overall, regular participants in even vigorous exercise, including those with established CHD, carry a considerably reduced risk of adverse events. Certainly, after myocardial infarction, active exercise rehabilitation has been shown to promote recovery and reduce subsequent mortality.

Advice on recommended exercises must be practical and realistic, tailored to the medical and social conditions of the patients. Many elderly patients have varying degrees of osteoarthritis, which limits

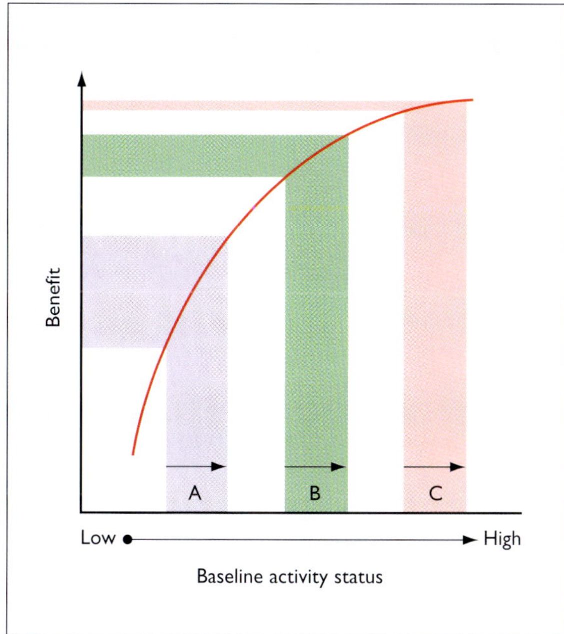

Figure 8.7. Estimated dose–response relationship between physical activity and health benefit. A, sedentary; B, moderately active; C, active. The lower the baseline physical activity status, the greater will be the health benefit associated with a given rise in physical activity (arrows A, B and C). After Pate *et al* [15].

weight-bearing exercises. Swimming is often an excellent alternative for these patients, and many swimming pools allocate specific times for use by the elderly. An exercise bicycle (placed in front of the television to avoid boredom) is a useful option for those who cannot go outside easily or safely. Other alternatives include television programmes and videos that lead aerobics sessions. One useful pamphlet suitable for patients is *Exercise: Why Bother?* [16].

Exercise must be convenient for the individual, otherwise it is unlikely to be sustained in the long term. Sports and leisure centres increasingly run fitness and training programmes appropriate for different age groups.

Drug therapy

Assuming a suitable period of assessment (between 3 weeks and 6 months – the duration being inversely related to the severity of the

BP readings) and that non-pharmacological measures have been attempted and found to be insufficient, the national and international management guidelines [2–6] are in agreement regarding the following general issues relating to drug therapy:

- Either systolic or diastolic BP criteria for treatment should be considered.
- Drug therapy should be considered at least up to the age of 80 years (trials above this age are in progress).
- Early and/or urgent treatment of severe and/or malignant hypertension.
- Thresholds for drug intervention should be lower for those with other major cardiovascular risk factors than among those without such risk factors.
- BP lowering regimens should attempt to reach specified targets.

When to treat

It is clear from trial evidence that important clinical benefits accrue from treating systolic BP ≥160 mmHg or diastolic BP ≥100 mmHg. Evidence for the benefits of treating lower levels of BP is less clear. Nevertheless, on the basis of prospective data such as those shown in Table 5.1 and Figure 5.1, current guidelines recommend that thresholds for intervention are lowered for patients with target organ damage, established vascular disease, diabetes or those above certain estimated levels of coronary or cardiovascular risk. Consequently, various risk assessment charts (Figs 8.8–8.11;Table 8.5a,b) have been developed to facilitate this approach of identifying hypertension in patients.

Absolute risk scores

While absolute risk of cardiovascular disease is more accurately evaluated by one of the recently produced computerized systems [17], use of one of the risk charts (Figs 8.9, 8.10) for men and women is a simple alternative. As can be seen, these charts provide a sex-specific, 5- or 10-year estimate of risk of a cardiovascular or coronary event based on data for several risk factors (diabetes, smoking, total cholesterol, HDL cholesterol, systolic BP, diastolic BP and age). These charts are recommended as a useful tool for motivating patients to change lifestyle and to aid the physician in evaluating risk levels and for treatment decision-making. A further simplification of the New Zealand or Joint British Recommendation charts is given in Figure 8.11, the use of which demands that patients with diabetes be considered as if they have active vascular disease (i.e. as in secondary prevention).

Finally, a simpler still, but therefore slightly less accurate, method of quantifying cardiovascular risk is the approach of counting risk factors and classifying hypertensive patients on that basis is shown in Tables 8.5a, b. The treatment algorithm in the most recent BHS guidelines which incorporated estimation of absolute risk (by whatever means) is shown in Figure 8.12.

TARGET

Concern is occasionally expressed that there may be a downside to lowering BP too far, as this produces a J-shaped association between BP lowering and mortality (Fig. 8.13). While it may be that in certain subgroups, perhaps those with active CHD and/or marked LVH, a J-shaped effect does occur, the evidence for this is limited. On the other hand, in the Systolic Hypertension in Elderly Program (SHEP) study [18], in which isolated systolic hypertension was treated with a diuretic or placebo, average diastolic BP in the actively treated group fell to <68 mmHg. It is more than likely that a large proportion of those actively treated had at least subclinical CHD. Nevertheless, both stroke and coronary benefits were associated with active treatment in this trial. Similarly in the many heart failure trials in which BP tends to start low, the use of drugs that also lower BP (usually ACE inhibitors) have been associated with highly significant reductions in coronary events and death. Consequently, by and large, concerns about 'overtreatment' and a 'J-effect' appear to be misplaced. Current recommendations for target BP based mainly on evidence from the HOT trial are shown in Table 8.6

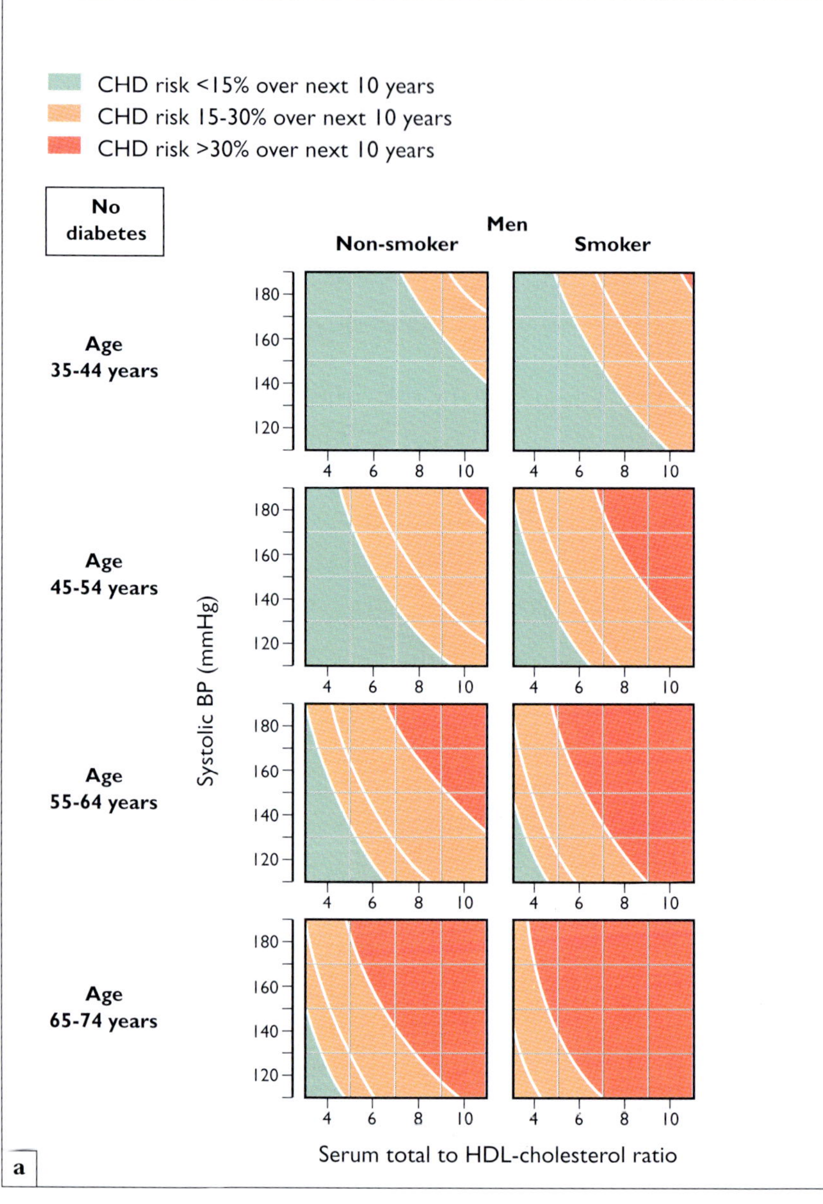

Figure 8.8 (a). Joint British societies coronary risk prediction charts for men. The chart should not be used for predicting risk in patients with coronary or

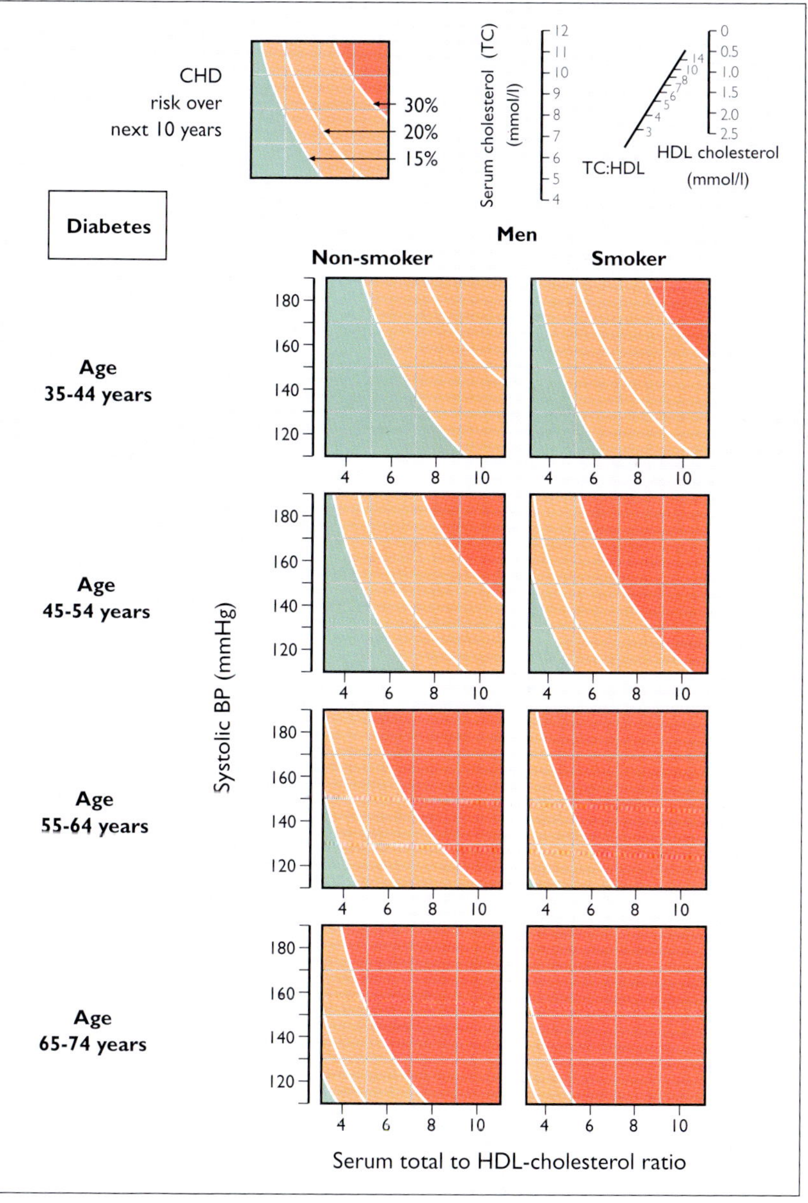

other major atherosclerotic disease, familial hypercholesterolaemia or those with renal failure.

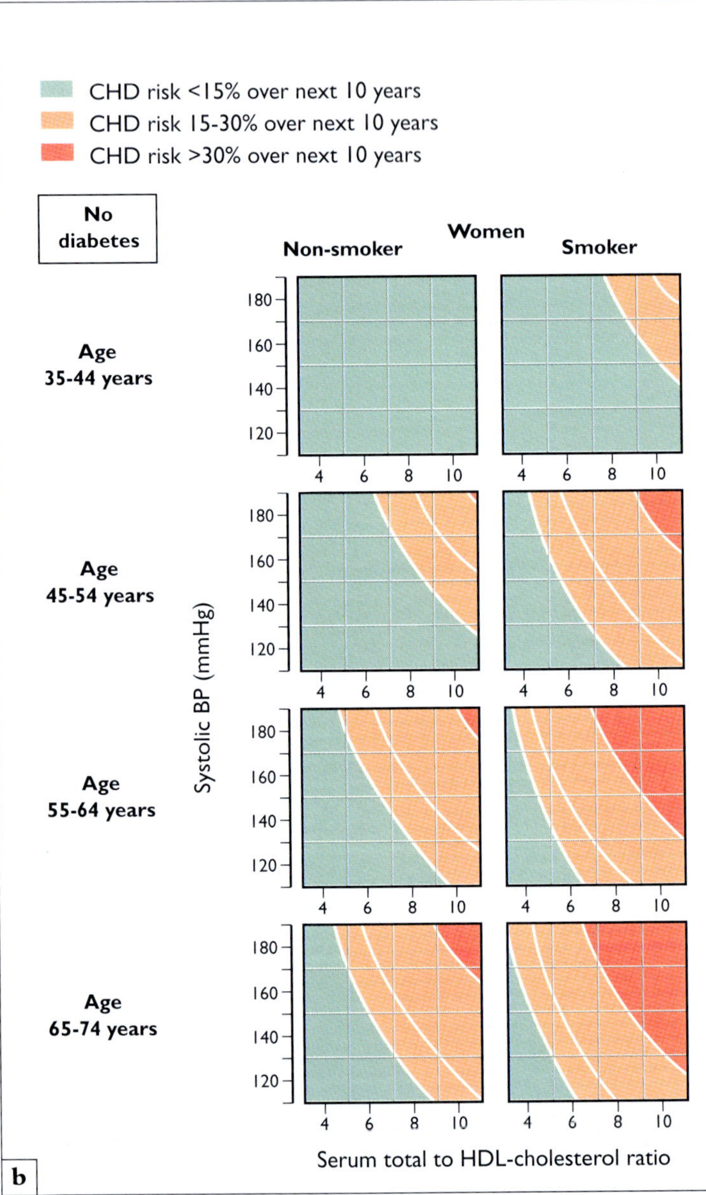

Figure 8.8 (b). Joint British societies coronary risk prediction charts for women. The chart should not be used for predicting risk in women with

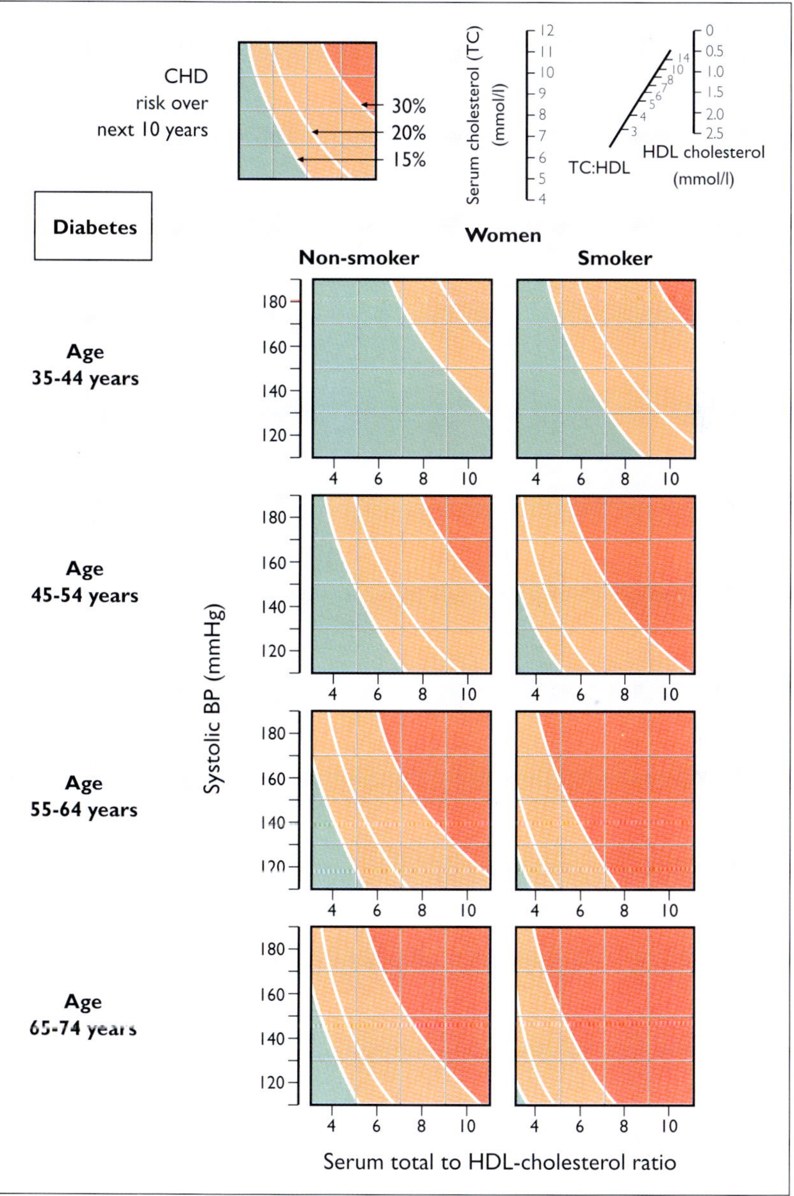

coronary or other major atherosclerotic disease, familial hypercholesterolaemia or those with renal failure.

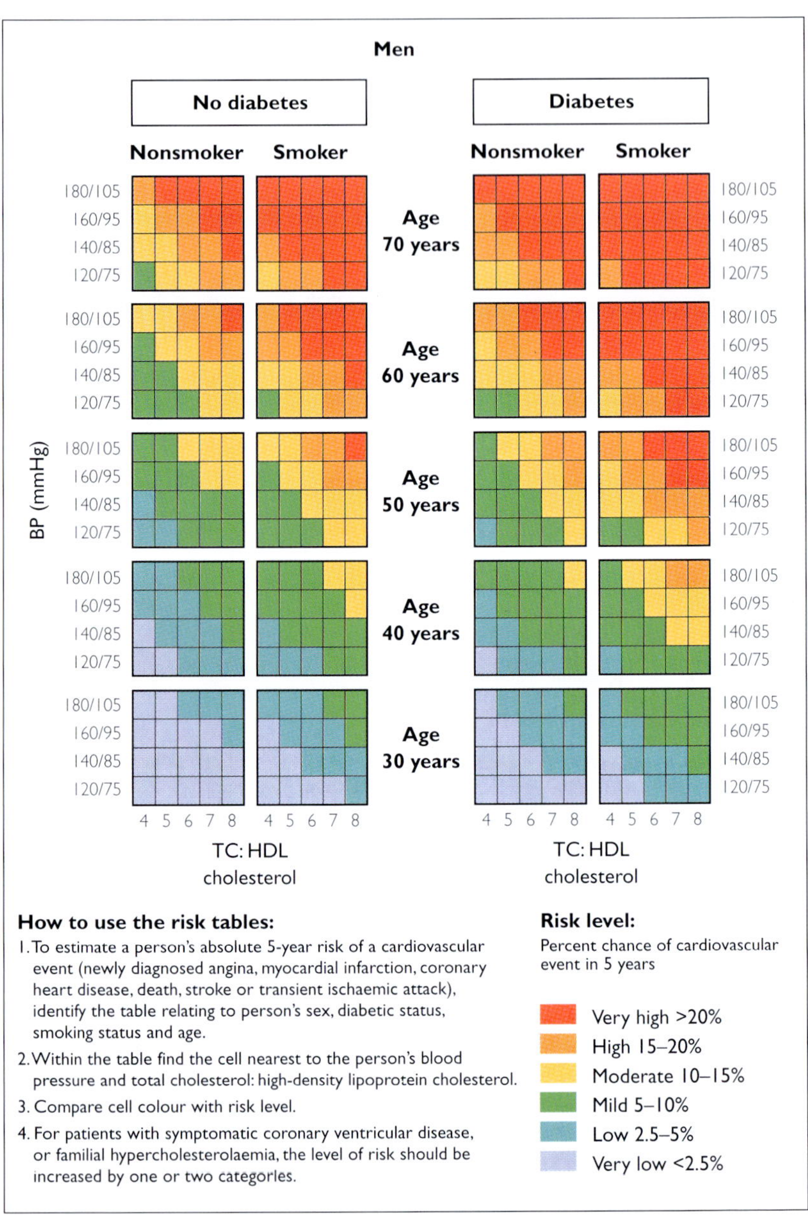

Figure 8.9. Estimating risk of a cardiovascular or coronary event based on data on several risk factors (men).

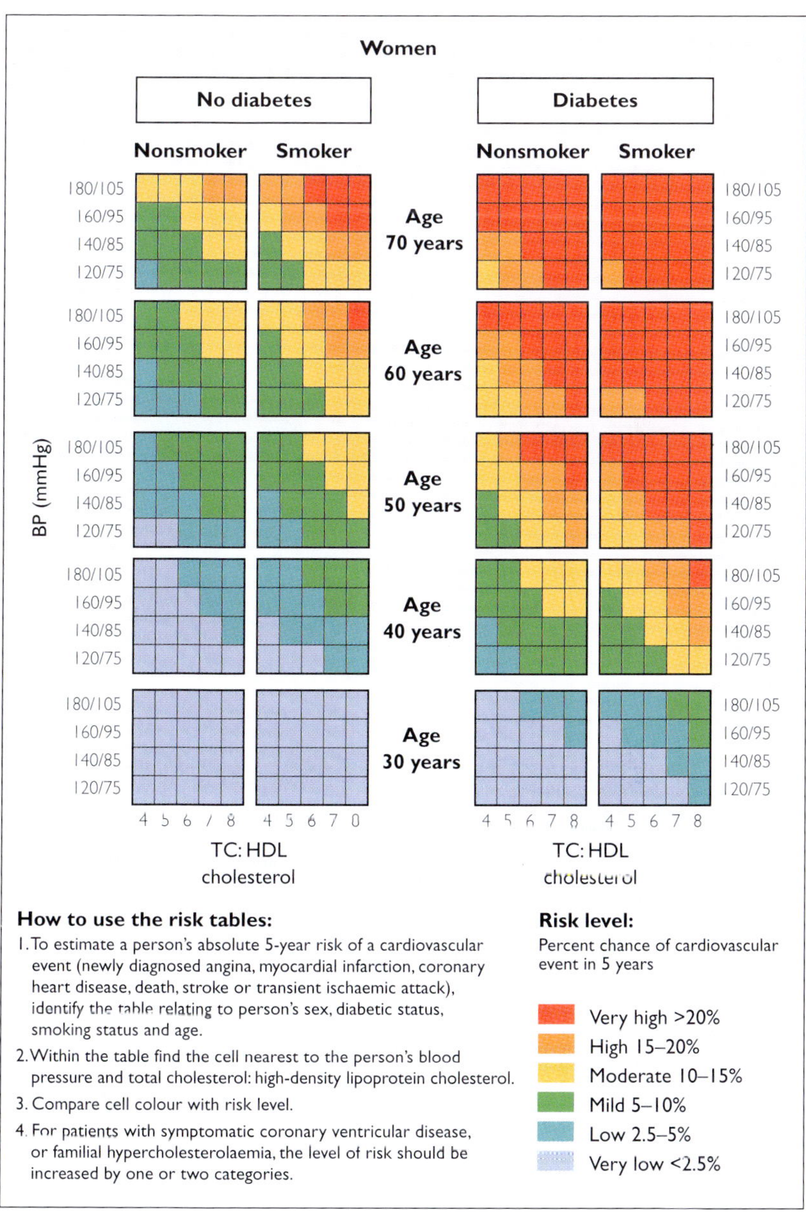

Figure 8.10. Estimating risk of a cardiovascular or coronary event based on data on several risk factors (women).

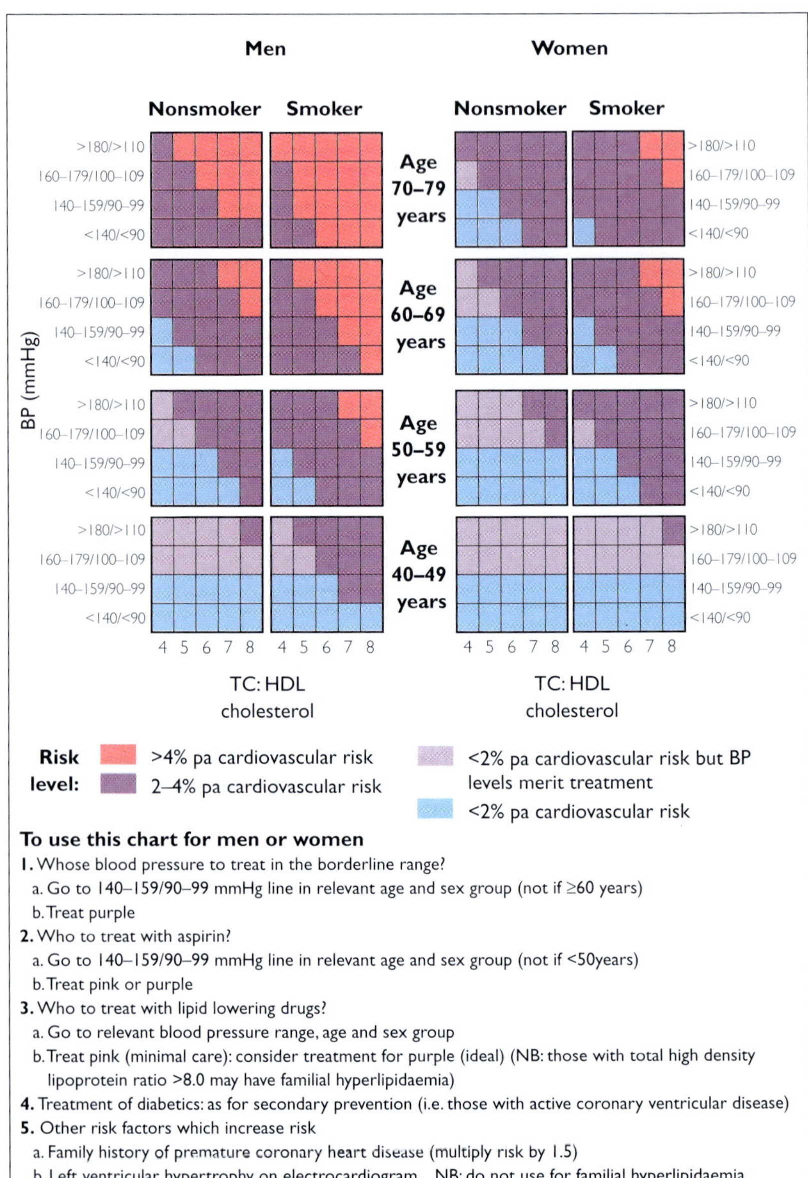

Figure 8.11. A further simplification of the New Zealand or Joint British Recommendation charts.

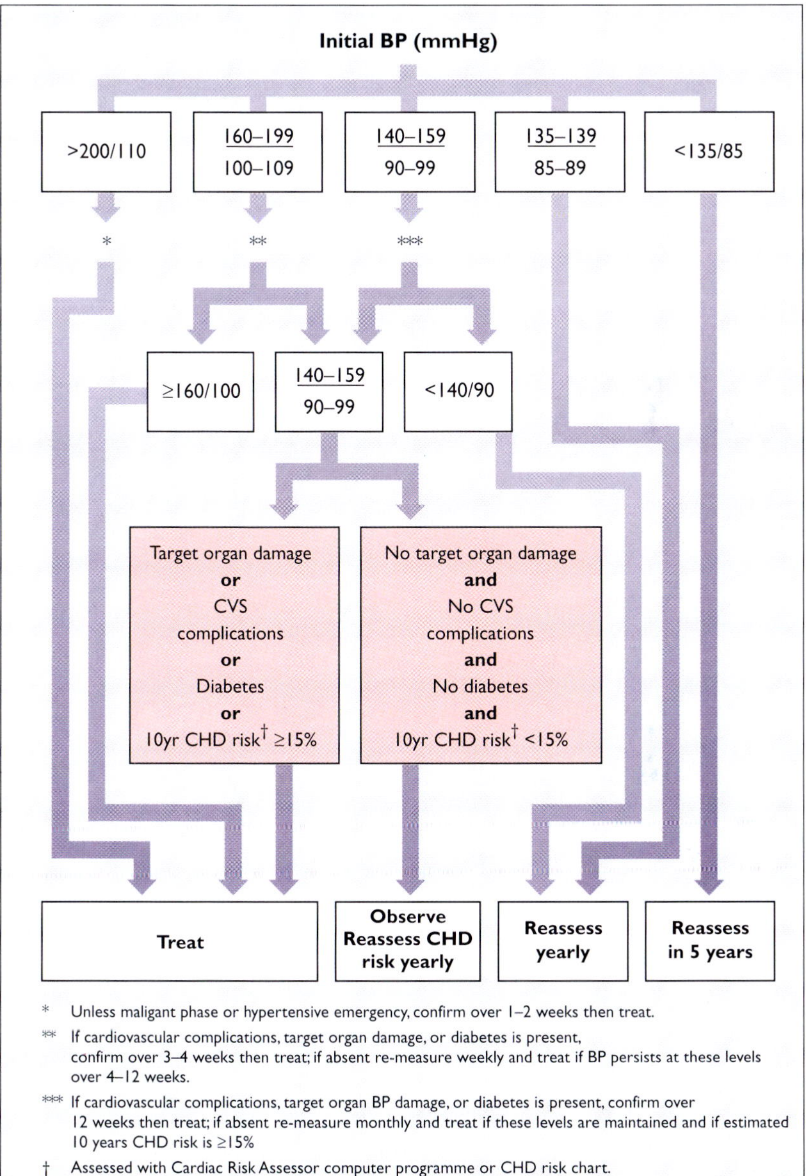

Figure 8.12. Treatment based on BP.

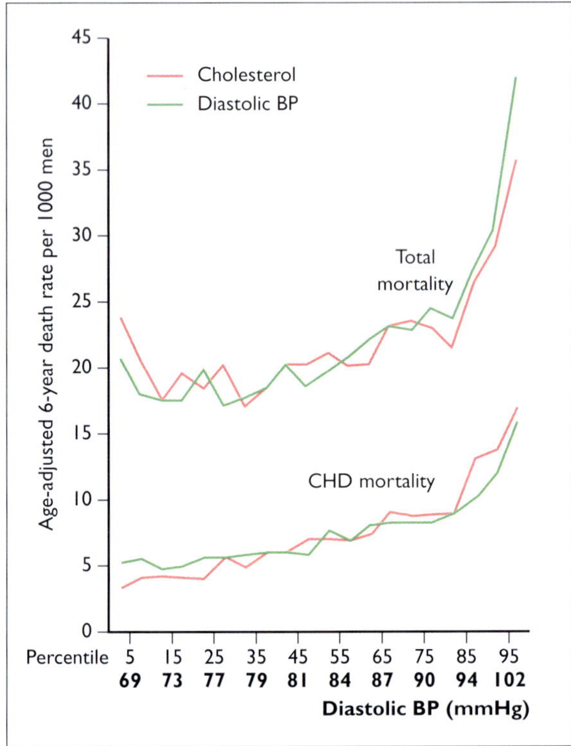

Figure 8.13. Age-adjusted CHD and total 6-year death rate per 1000 men screened for the Multiple Risk Factor Intervention Trial according to diastolic BP and cholesterol centiles.

Which drugs?

Most of the national and international guidelines recommend that drug therapy should be initiated with a diuretic or β-blocker, assuming these drugs are not contraindicated or there are compelling reasons for the use of other agents. The rationale for this recommendation is that in almost all of the long-term morbidity and mortality trials hitherto, these were the two principal drug groups used.

The most recent guidelines from America (Joint National Committee VI [JNC VI]) [4], the World Health Organization –International Society of Hypertension (WHO–ISH) Consensus

Table 8.5a. Risk stratification and treatment*

BP stages (mmHg)	Risk Group A (no risk factors; no TOD/CCD†)	Risk Group B (at least 1 risk factor, not including diabetes; no TOD/CCD)	Risk Group C (TOD/CCD and/or diabetes, with or without other risk factors)
High–normal (130–139/ 85–89)	Lifestyle modification	Lifestyle modification	Drug therapy‡
Stage 1 (140–159/ 90–99)	Lifestyle modification (up to 12 months)	Lifestyle modification§ (up to 6 months)	Drug therapy
Stages 2 and 3 (≥160/≥100)	Drug therapy	Drug therapy	Drug therapy

* Note: for example, a patient with diabetes and a BP of 142/94 mmHg plus LVH should be classified as having Stage 1 hypertension with target organ disease (LVH) and with another major risk factor (diabetes). This patient would be categorized as 'Stage 1, Risk Group C', and recommended immediate initiation of pharmacological treatment. Lifestyle modification should be adjunctive therapy for all patients recommended for pharmacological therapy.

†TOD/CCD, target organ disease/clinical cardiovascular disease (see Table 8.5b).

‡For those with heart failure, renal insufficiency or diabetes.

§For patients with multiple risk factors, clinicians should consider drugs as the initial therapy plus lifestyle modification (see Table 8.5b).

Table 8.5b. Components of cardiovascular risk stratification in patients with hypertension

Major risk factors

- Smoking
- Dyslipidaemia
- Diabetes mellitus
- Age >60 years
- Sex (men and postmenopausal women)
- Family history of cardiovascular disease: women <65 years or men <55 years

Target organ damage/clinical cardiovascular disease

- Heart diseases:
  LVH
  angina or prior myocardial infarction
  prior coronary revascularization
  heart failure
- Stroke or transient ischaemic attack
- Nephropathy
- Peripheral arterial disease
- Retinopathy

Group [5] and the British Hypertension Society (BHS) [6], while acknowledging that most trial data relate to diuretics and that these are the cheapest agents available, have all moved towards the approach of tailoring treatment to the individual profile of the patient. The rationale for this approach is based on both therapeutic and mechanistic considerations.

Therapeutic considerations

- The prognosis of hypertensives is greatly influenced by the presence of other risk factors (which commonly coexist with hypertension) and by target organ damage (Chapter 6).

Table 8.6. Suggested target BP during antihypertensive treatment. Systolic *and* diastolic should both be attained (e.g. <140/85 mmHg means <140 mmHg systolic *and* <85 mmHg diastolic)

	Clinic BP		Mean day-time ambulatory BP or home BP	
	No diabetes	Diabetes	No diabetes	Diabetes
Optimal BP	<140/85	< 140/80	<130/80	<130/75
Audit standard*	<150/90	<140/85	< 140/85	<140/80

*The audit standard reflects the minimum recommended levels of BP control.

Despite best practice, the audit standard is not achievable in all treated hypertensives.

- Different drug groups exert differential effects on the frequently coexistent risk factors and target organ damage.
- Trial-based evidence has expanded recently (see Chapter 12) and newer agents have been shown to be at least as effective as diuretics or β-blockers in certain types of patients.

Hence, even pending further long-awaited, long-term morbidity and mortality trial data on newer agents, there seems a cogent argument to individualize therapy on the basis of certain risk factor and target organ profiles. Factors that might influence drug choice are given in Table 8.7.

Mechanistic considerations

It is most unlikely that hypertension is the result of a single pathological process. While the cellular and molecular mechanisms that underlie the pathogenetic process have not been identified, it appears, from the available evidence, that a multiplicity of environmental and genetic factors may contribute to BP elevation in the population at large (Fig.

Table 8.7. Factors that may influence initial choice of drug therapy

- Lifestyle
- Age
- Sex
- Race
- Lipids
- Diabetes
- Coronary heart disease (angina, heart failure)
- LVF
- Coexisting disease, e.g. asthma, gout, intermittent claudication

4.11). Similarly, it seems unlikely a single preferred drug will cover the broad spectrum of people with hypertension, any more than one antibiotic can be used for all types of infections.

Advantages, disadvantages and common side effects

The advantages, disadvantages and common side effects of the six main drug classes are shown in Table 8.8, and some examples of patient profiling, as suggested in the most recent BHS and WHO–ISH guidelines, are shown in Table 8.9.

Looking to the future it seems reasonable that the use of low doses of two currently available agents in combination may become a preferred first-line therapeutic approach. This approach has the potential advantage of producing at least additive, and in certain cases synergistic, effects on BP lowering, while at the same time, because of the low doses used, it results in fewer side-effects and so increased tolerability and compliance, and hence greater efficacy. Table 8.10 shows some logical and some less logical combinations.

Table 8.8. Advantages, disadvantages and side effects of drug treatments

Treatment	Advantages	Disadvantages	Side effects
Diuretics	Low cost Effective in elderly	↓K^+, leading to arrhythmias ↑glucose ↑cholesterol and triglycerides ↑uric acid	Impotence Urinary frequency Gout
β-blockers	Good for angina Good for anxiety Good for post MI	↑triglycerides ↓HDL cholesterol ↓cardiac output/exercise tolerance Contraindicated in asthma; caution in CCF and PVD	Lethargy Raynaud's phenomenon Sleep disturbance Depression Impotence
ACE inhibitors	LVH regression ↓Na^+ retention Lipid neutral Renal protection in diabetes	Contraindicated in renal artery stenosis and women of child-bearing potential	Cough Hypotension (with diuretic)
AII antagonists	Well tolerated (no 'ACE' cough)	As for ACE inhibitors	Hypotension (with diuretic)
Calcium antagonists	Lipid neutral Weak diuretic effect Anti-anginal effect	Negative inotropic effect of verapamil and diltiazem Short-acting drugs contraindicated in CHD	Flushing Headaches Oedema
α-blockers	Improve lipid profile and insulin resistance Improve sexual potency Improve prostatism	Caution in heart failure	Palpitations Postural hypotension (with short-acting agents)

Table 8.9. Compelling and possible indications, contraindications and cautions for the major classes of antihypertensive drugs

Class of drug	Compelling indications	Possible indications	Possible contraindications	Compelling contraindications
α-blockers	Prostatism	Dyslipidaemia Sexual dysfunction	Postural hypotension Heart failure	Urinary incontinence
ACE inhibitors	Heart failure Left ventricular dysfunction Type 1 diabetic neuropathy	Chronic renal disease* Type 2 diabetic neuropathy	Renal impairment* PVD+	Pregnancy Renovascular disease
AII-antagonists	ACE inhibitor-induced‡ cough	Heart failure Intolerance of other antihypertensive drugs	PVD+	Pregnancy Renovascular disease
β-blockers	Myocardial infarction Angina	Heart failure§	Heart failure§ Dyslipidaemia PVD	Asthma/COPD Heart block
Calcium antagonists (dihydropyridine)	Elderly ISH	Elderly Angina	–	–
Calcium antagonists (rate-limiting)	Angina	Myocardial infarction	Combination with β-blockade	Heart block Heart failure
Thiazides	Elderly ISH Heart failure		Dyslipidaemia	Gout

* ACE inhibitors may be beneficial in chronic renal failure, but should only be used with caution Close supervision and specialist advice is required when there is established and significant renal impairment.

+ Caution with ACE inhibitors and AII antagonists in PVD because of association with renovascular disease.

‡ If ACE inhibitor indicated.

§ β-blockers may worsen heart failure, but in specialist hands may be used to treat heart failure.

Current status of hypertension management

Treatment rates among English adults with hypertension (defined as a systolic BP ≥160 mmHg, diastolic BP ≥95 mmHg or on treatment for hypertension) evaluated in a 1994 survey [19] are shown in Table 8.11. The proportion of these hypertensives whose BP was controlled using a conservative definition of systolic BP <160 mmHg and diastolic BP <95 mmHg is also shown in Table 8.11.

Table 8.10. Logical and less logical agent combinations

Logical drug combinations

- Diuretic and β-blocker
- Diuretic and ACE inhibitor
- Dihydropyridine calcium antagonist and β-blocker
- Calcium antagonist and ACE-inhibitor
- α-blocker and β-blocker
- ACE inhibitor and α-blocker

Less logical combinations

- Calcium antagonist and diuretic
- β-blocker and ACE inhibitor

Beware

- Rate-limiting calcium antagonist (e.g. verapamil, diltiazem) and β-blocker

Table 8.11. Treatment and control of BP among English adults with hypertension [19]

	Patients	Treatment (%)	Control (%)
Men	1044	45	27
Women	1315	55	32
All	2359	51	30

It is clear that overall in 1994 more than two-thirds of hypertensives in England had uncontrolled BP, even using these conservative criteria for 'control'. It is reassuring that this proportion has fallen more recently but even today the majority are 'uncontrolled', by this definition.

A similar proportion of hypertensives are 'uncontrolled' in the USA, but the proportion in the USA relates to a definition of hypertension and control of 140/90 mmHg. Therefore, in England (the situation is likely to be similar or worse in the rest of the UK), the hypertensive population's BP is about 20/5 mmHg higher than that in the USA. This is reflected in lower death rates for stroke and CHD in the USA.

The majority (60%) of hypertensive patients on treatment currently receive one drug to lower BP, with 34% and 6% receiving two and three or more drugs, respectively. Among those who receive one drug, the most commonly prescribed agents are as shown in Table 8.12; in Table 8.13 the most commonly used combinations of drugs are shown. It is of interest that the second most common combination of drugs (calcium antagonists plus diuretics) is not considered to be a very effective pairing in terms of BP lowering.

IDEAL REQUIREMENTS OF ANTIHYPERTENSIVE AGENTS

The ultimate requirement of an antihypertensive regimen is that it should provide optimal prevention of the adverse cardiovascular events attributable to elevated arterial pressure.

To achieve this, the regimen should lower BP effectively and prevent and/or reverse target organ damage and vascular remodelling induced by hypertension. In addition, since the aetiology of cardiovascular disease is multifactorial, antihypertensive agents should, ideally, not adversely affect any of the other risk factors for cardiovascular disease. As compliance is critically dependent upon drug tolerability, one further prerequisite for the practical efficacy of any antihypertensive agent is that it should be well tolerated. Finally, given the financial restrictions prevalent in health budgets worldwide, antihypertensive management must be cost-effective.

Table 8.12. Types of drug being ingested by those being administered one drug for hypertension [19]

All ages (*n* = 707)	Use (%)
Diuretic	36
β-blocker	29
Calcium antagonist	22
Angiotensin-converting enzyme inhibitor	11
Other	2

Table 8.13. Most common treatment combinations used for hypertension [19]

Combination	Use (%)
Diuretic + β-blocker	41
Diuretic + calcium antagonist	19
Diuretic + ACE inhibitor	12
β-blocker + calcium antagonist	12
ACE inhibitor + calcium antagonist	4
Others	12

Dealing with each of these issues in the context of currently available agents, the meta-analyses of the intervention trials suggest a shortfall in CHD prevention associated with the use of diuretics and β-blockers [20]. This controversial observation has been attributed to the failure of these two groups of drugs to satisfy two of the other ideal requirements of antihypertensive agents mentioned above, namely the ability to prevent or reverse various forms of target organ damage and compatibility with a multiple risk-factor approach to management. Some of the newer classes of agents – ACE inhibitors, angiotensin II (AII) receptor antagonists, α-blockers and calcium antagonists – appear to offer advantages in these areas, although these agents as yet remain relatively unevaluated in long-term morbidity and mortality trials compared with diuretics and β-blockers.

All the major drug groups currently in use appear, when used in equivalent doses, to be similarly effective in terms of BP lowering, although some drugs may be more or less effective in different types of patient [21]. However, in the randomized controlled trials of hypertension management, the mean reduction in diastolic BP was only 5–6 mmHg. In clinical practice, all agents are likely to be more effective at preventing cardiovascular disease if greater falls in BP are achieved, as suggested by prospective observational data [22], and at least in subgroups of patients by data from two recently published trials [23,24].

The Treatment of Mild Hypertension Study (TOMHS) [25], which is the only study to date to compare five major drug groups in a long-term trial, demonstrated a similar frequency of side effects in patients, whether they took a β-blocker, calcium antagonist, diuretic, ACE inhibitor or α-blocker. Hence, with regard to tolerability, there appears to be little quantitative difference between the various antihypertensive agents currently in common use. Equally important, however, is that side effects were reported less frequently by those on active drug therapy than by those on placebo. While this is encouraging, rates of withdrawal of participants from the major hypertension trials range from 20% to over 50%. It is also clear that, in practice, poor compliance, again critically influenced by side-effect rates, is currently a major problem in the hypertensive population. Current early evidence suggests that AII antagonists may offer an advantage over other drug groups in this regard.

Much of the focus regarding the cost efficacy of various antihypertensive agents has been placed on the relative costs of available drugs, and the differences are undoubtedly large. However, in evaluating any policy for intervention on health, the benefits should also be considered. Until all available agents have been evaluated in the long-term morbidity and mortality trials in progress [26], to compare 'benefits' only 'surrogate' end-points such as regression of LVH are available. It may be that cheaper agents are not the most cost effective.

Methods for improving cardiovascular risk among hypertensive patients are summarized in Table 8.14. It seems likely that the improved prevention of cardiovascular disease by hypertension management can most easily be achieved by better BP control. The first step towards reaching this goal is to follow the recommendations for thresholds and goals for intervention outlined in any of the national and international guidelines [2–6]. However, in practice, better BP control for those patients on therapy can only be achieved if drug tolerability and hence compliance are not reduced as drug doses are increased. Looking to the future, it is possible that more effective agents with fewer side effects

Table 8.14. Cardiovascular risk reduction: how to do better for hypertensives
Improve BP control
Follow guidelines
Ensure 24-hour control
Population strategy
?Low-dose combinations (unproven as yet)
Reduce drug side effects
Non-pharmacological therapy
New drugs
?Low-dose combinations (unproven as yet)
Increase focused prescribing
Address other risk factors
More accurate risk prediction
Exclude white-coat hypertension
Pre-empt and /or reverse target organ damage

will be developed. Alternatively, as mentioned above, the use of low doses of two currently available agents in combination may, as a preferred 'first-line' approach, increase tolerability and compliance.

Finally, through more accurate identification of those at increased risk – perhaps by noninvasive direct visualization of vessels and target organs – more accurate targeting of resources and therapy will produce more effective prevention of cardiovascular disease.

THE PLACE OF AUDIT IN HYPERTENSION (Fig. 8.14)

We have seen the recent development and dissemination of various national and international guidelines on the management of hypertension [5,6]. The aim of these guidelines is to put forward programmes to allow the correct identification and management of hypertension in the community and to reduce the possible adverse effects of any hypertensive treatment. The guidelines give clear indications for management decisions and lend themselves to the audit process. Management requires a multidisciplinary approach, which entails careful BP measurement, regular review and recognition that different treatments have different limitations and side effects that may affect quality of life and compliance. A summary of guidelines (Table 8.15) is provided by BHS [6].

It is suggested that all practices or primary care groups should develop a protocol for hypertension management that covers:

- Screening policy
- Initial evaluation and investigation
- Implementation of non-pharmacological measures
- Formal estimation of cardiovascular risk
- Treatment policy for antihypertensive drugs, aspirin and statins
- Treatment targets
- Policy for follow-up and methods for identifying and recalling patients who drop out of follow-up.

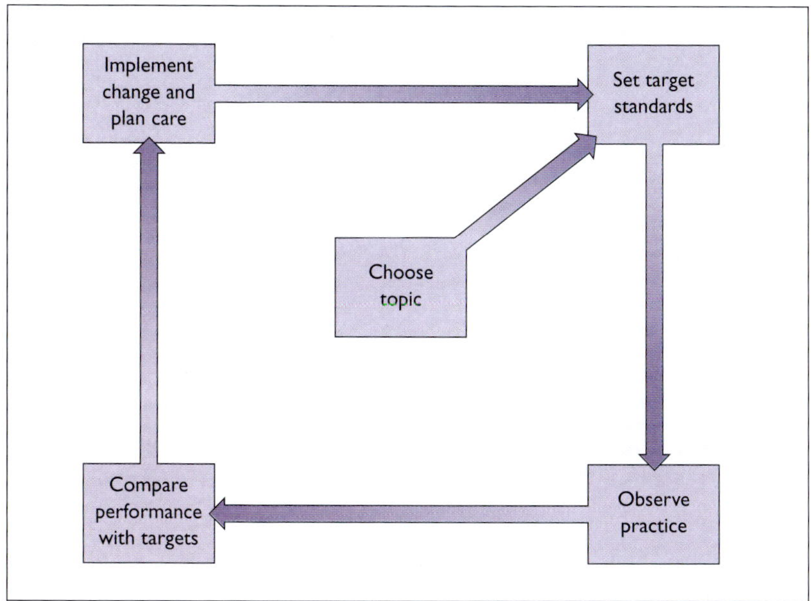

Figure 8.14. The Audit Cycle.

Written information should be available for patients about hypertension and its treatment, and about non-pharmacological measures to reduce BP and cardiovascular risk. Practice policy should detail those aspects of management that are in the province of the practice nurse and of the doctor, as well as the indications and procedure for passing management from nurse to doctor or vice versa.

Audit activity needs to be simple and focused on specific terms of reference as a means of making sure we provide optimum care to our patients. It is a necessary and invaluable part of patient care and should praise achievement as well as being constructively critical. Feedback and re-audit is necessary to ensure that any agreed recommendations are implemented and effective.

Table 8.15. Guidelines for hypertension management

- Use non-pharmacological measures in all hypertensives and borderline hypertensives.
- Initiate antihypertensive drug therapy in patients with sustained systolic BP ≥160 mmHg or sustained diastolic BP ≥100 mmHg.
- Decide on treatment in patients with sustained systolic BP between 140 and 159 mmHg or sustained diastolic BP between 90 and 99 mmHg according to the presence or absence of target organ damage, cardiovascular disease or a 10-year CHD risk of ≥15% according to the Joint British Societies CHD risk assessment programme or risk chart.
- In patients with diabetes mellitus, initiate antihypertensive drug therapy if systolic BP is sustained at ≥140 mmHg or diastolic BP is sustained at ≥90 mmHg.
- In nondiabetic hypertensives, optimal BP targets are a systolic BP <140 mmHg and a diastolic BP <85 mmHg. The minimum acceptable level of control (audit standard) recommended is <150/<90 mmHg. Despite best practice, these levels are difficult to achieve in some hypertensives.
- In diabetic hypertensives, optimal BP targets are a systolic BP <140 mmHg and a diastolic BP <80 mmHg. The minimum acceptable level of control (audit standard) recommended is <140/<85 mmHg. Despite best practice, these levels are difficult to achieve in some patients with diabetes and hypertension.
- In the absence of contraindications or compelling indications for other antihypertensive agents, low-dose thiazide diuretics or β-blockers are preferred as first-line therapy for the majority of hypertensives. In the absence of compelling indications for β-blockade, diuretics or long-acting dihydropyridine calcium anti-antagonists are preferred to β-blockers in older subjects.

  Compelling indications and contraindications for all antihypertensive drug classes are specified in Table 8.9.
- For most hypertensives, a combination of antihypertensive drugs is required to achieve the recommended targets for BP control.

Table 8.15. (continued)

- Other drugs that reduce cardiovascular risk must also be considered. These include aspirin for secondary prevention of cardiovascular disease, and for primary prevention in treated hypertensives over the age of 50 years who have a 10-year CHD risk ≥15% and in whom BP is controlled to the audit standard. In accordance with existing British guidelines, statin therapy is recommended for hypertensives with a TC ≥5 mmol/l and established vascular disease, or a 10-year CHD risk ≥30% estimated from the Joint British Societies CHD risk chart. Glycaemic control should also be optimized in diabetic subjects.
- Specific advice is given on the management of hypertension in specific patient groups (see Chapters 9 and 10), that is the elderly, ethnic subgroups, diabetes mellitus, chronic renal disease and in females (pregnancy, oral contraceptive use and hormone replacement therapy).

The first essential step towards effective audit is to approach it in a positive way: 'Am I, or are we, doing well?' and 'Can I, or can we, do better?' Audit should involve staff as well as the doctors and is a collective way of improving patient care. Staff who carry out the audit should be team members and should attend meetings to discuss the results. It is important to have a clear purpose in mind and to ask simple questions – keep it short and simple [27].

What can audit evaluate?

The primary health-care team (PHCT) may choose to audit any aspects of the management of the hypertensive patient listed in Table 8.16. In the UK, the National Service Framework document published in 2000 provides evidence-based and explicit information on the management of cardiovascular patients. There are some helpful audit protocols available as part of this document. For example:

- *Completeness of the arterial disease, cerebrovascular disease and hypertension registers* – by comparison with published prevalence and by cross checks with diagnostic codes
- *Recording of risk factors and levels of control in patients* – including smoking, BP, BMI, physical activity and cholesterol
- *Clinic attendance* – plus the number of patients on the register not seen for more than 12 months
- *Prescribing rates* – for aspirin and lipid-lowering drugs
- *Screening* – proportions of the population, categorised by sex and ten-year age groups, recording:
    - BP
    - Smoking
    - Significant family history

Table 8.16. What can audit evaluate?

- The proportion of all adults who have had BP measurement in past 5 years.
- Urinalysis checked at diagnosis and subsequently.
- How many BP measurements were taken before the treatment was initiated?
- At each visit were two BP measurements taken?
- How many patients with hypertension have been identified and are receiving treatment?
- Were the following points in the history identified?
    - smoking
    - alcohol
    - medication
    - exercise
    - current history of CHD
    - past history of CHD
    - diabetes mellitus

Table 8.16. (continued)

HRT or contraceptive method used
respiratory illness, especially asthma or COPD
family history of CHD
history of cerebrovascular disease

- Were the following examinations and investigations performed during the first month of diagnosis?
  body weight
  urinalysis
  fundoscopy
  femoral pulses checked
  palpation of kidneys
  auscultation for renal and carotid bruits
  signs of LVH
  tests of renal function
  blood lipids
  blood glucose
  uric acid
  ECG
- Does the practice have management guidelines, checklists, computer support, patient held record cards and patient information leaflets?
  What proportion of patients were given non-pharmacological advice?
  What proportion of patients have suboptimal control?
  What proportion of patients are lost to follow-up or not reviewed in previous 6 months?
- What is the use of aspirin and statins by those who require secondary prevention, or their use when indicated for primary prevention (i.e. when the estimated 10-year CHD is ≥15% (aspirin) or ≥30% per year (statin)? (See Chapter 8)
  What proportion of patients meet targets set for lipid levels?
  Have enquiries been made regarding side effects?

There will be a review of this protocol in approximately two years' time, once new and relevant guidelines have been published

Pharmacological management of these patients could be examined with specific regard to the use of practice protocols and guidelines. The objective of this approach is to make the treating physician aware of any deviation from the guidelines, thus enabling review of current practice and treatment.

Choose a specific target group

An important question to answer before embarking on an audit is 'How big should the sample be?' If it is too small, it might be unrepresentative or misleading, and if it is too large, it may waste practice time and resources. Decide on how much data you wish to collect. A small sample may be adequate for a pilot study to give a general impression; however, a larger, more reliable and more representative sample gives a much more realistic measure of the group's performance. In an ideal world we should audit all patients in the target group and this may be possible in small practices. However, in a larger practice a sample that is representative of the whole group of hypertensive patients is needed, ideally chosen by random selection.

Experience has shown that very few practices have all their patient data on the computer in a way that enables a comprehensive search to be performed and inevitably note pulling is necessary.

How to choose your sample

Personal sampling

Comparisons may be made within a practice by personal sampling techniques, but such a sample is likely to be unrepresentative.

Random sampling

The use of random sampling means that each hypertensive patient has an equal chance of being selected. All patients are given a number starting from 1, and then selected using a random number generator.

Systematic sampling

For example, if we choose 350 hypertensives out of a total of 5000, every fourteenth patient on the list is audited. Systematic sampling like this may lead to some undetected source of bias and care needs to be taken if this method is chosen. The starting point should be chosen at random. Computer generated lists are usually in alphabetical order and it is necessary to rearrange the names in a different sequence to avoid bias.

Stratified sampling

Stratified sampling involves splitting the patients into groups such as age, sex, type of treatment, etc., and then using random selection or systematic sampling from within each group.

Cluster sampling

Cluster sampling involves selecting a sample of groups (cluster) instead of sampling from each of the individual groups. This method is unlikely to be representative of the whole group but may be useful if one particular member of the partnership wishes to look at his or her own individual performance.

Criteria

The criteria must be chosen to match the advice given by the guidelines, whether international, national or local. If the standard is set at 100%, disappointment is inevitable.

Steps to carry out an audit

1. Discuss the audit among members of the PHCT and nominate a coordinator.
2. Agree on the aims and objectives of the audit and the process of data collection and analysis.
3. Identify the notes of all hypertensive patients in the target group. This may be achieved by means of a disease register, computer records or a repeat prescribing list.

4. Choose a suitable sample size, and decide on your sampling technique.
5. Scrutinize each set of notes or perform a computer search to determine the presence or absence of the required data and transfer this data onto a spreadsheet.
6. Agree on a reasonable timescale for completion of the data collection and analysis.
7. Compare performance with the standards.
8. Review the information and identify whether or not the standards have been met.

Agree and implement change

Arrange a meeting to discuss the results of the audit and decide what changes are necessary to enable the team to comply with the guidelines. The agreed changes should be monitored and the audit cycle completed after a suitable time lapse.

Chapter Summary

- Preventive strategies can be subdivided into high-risk strategy and population based.
- The majority of the preventive effort is currently directed towards the high-risk strategy.
- The alternative population approach is essentially an attempt to move the distribution of BP in the whole population downwards.
- Given the multifactorial aetiology of cardiovascular disease, the alteration of any one risk factor may produce only limited benefit.
- Lifestyle modification, particularly advice to stop smoking, is essential in all hypertensive patients, irrespective of severity.
- Treatment should be tailored to the individual profile of the patient (e.g. as recommended by the latest BHS guidelines).

- It is reasonable, cost permitting, to use low doses of two currently available agents in combination as a first-line therapeutic approach.
- The ultimate requirement of antihypertensive regimens is that they should provide optimal prevention of the adverse cardiovascular events attributable to elevated arterial pressure.
- Treatment should be well tolerated and cost effective.
- Follow the recommendations for thresholds and goals for intervention outlined in the national and international guidelines.
- Enquire about side effects of drugs at follow-up visits.
- Check compliance with therapy.
- Regular audit to review performance.

References

1. Rose G. *The Strategy of Preventive Medicine*. Oxford: Oxford University Press, 1992.
2. Myers MG, Carruthers SG, Leenen FHH, Haynes RB. Recommendations from the Canadian Hypertension Society Consensus Conference on the pharmacologic treatment of hypertension. *Can Med Assoc J* 1989; **140**: 1141–6.
3. Jackson R, Barham P, Bills J, *et al*. Management of raised blood pressure in New Zealand: a discussion document. *BMJ* 1993; **307**: 107–10.
4. Joint National Committee on Detection Evaluation and Treatment of High Blood Pressure. The sixth report of the Joint National Committee on Prevention, Detection, and Treatment of High Blood Pressure (JNC VI). *Arch Intern Med* 1997; **157**: 2413–46.
5. WHO–ISH. 1999 World Health Organization–International Society of Hypertension Guidelines for the Management of Hypertension. *Blood Pressure* 1999; **8**: 1–43.
6. Ramsay LE, Johnston GD, MacGregor GA, *et al*. Guidelines for Management of Hypertension: Report of the third working party of the British Hypertension Society. *J Hum Hypertens* 1999; **13**(9): 569–92.

7. Raw M, McNeill A, West R. Smoking cessation guidelines for health professionals. A guide to effective smoking cessation interventions for the health care system. *Thorax* 1998; **53**: S1–19.
8. Raw M, McNeill A, West R. Smoking cessation: evidence-based recommendations for the healthcare system. *BMJ* 1999; **318**: 182–5.
9. Ebrahim S, Davey-Smith G. Lowering blood pressure: a systematic review of sustained effects of non-pharmacological interventions. *J Public Health Med* 1998; **20**: 441–8.
10. Appel LJ, Moore TJ, Obarzanek E, *et al.*, for the DASH Collaborative Research Group. A clinical trial of the effects of dietary patterns on blood pressure. *N Engl J Med* 1997; **336**: 1117–24.
11. Klatsky AL, Friedman GD, Siegelaub AB, Gerard MJ. Alcohol consumption and blood pressure: Kaiser-Permanente Multiphasic Health Examination data. *N Engl J Med* 1977; **296**: 1194–200.
12. Law MR, Frost CD, Wald NJ. By how much does dietary salt reduction lower blood pressure? III Analysis of data from trials of salt reduction. *BMJ* 1991; **302**: 819–24.
13. Khaw KT, Barrett-Connor E. Dietary potassium and stroke-associated mortality. A 12-year prospective population study. *N Engl J Med* 1987; **316**: 235–40.
14. Jennings G, Nelson L, Nestel P, *et al.* The effects of changes in physical activity on major cardiovascular risk factors, hemodynamics, sympathetic function, and glucose utilization in man: a controlled study of four levels of activity. *Circulation* 1986; **73**: 30–40.
15. Pate RR, Pratt M, Blair SN, *et al.* Physical activity and public health. *JAMA* 1995; **273**: 402–7.
16. *Exercise – why bother?* London: Health Education Authority.
17. Wood D, Durrington P, Poulter N, McInnes G, Rees A, Wray R for the British Cardiac Society, British Hyperlipidaemia Association, British Hypertension Society, and British Diabetic Association. Joint British recommendations on prevention of coronary heart disease in clinical practice. *Heart* 1998; **80**: 51–529.
18. SHEP Cooperative Research Group. Prevention of stroke by antihypertensive drug treatment in older persons with isolated systolic hypertension. Final results of the Systolic Hypertension in the Elderly Program (SHEP). *JAMA* 1991; **265**: 3255–64.
19. Colhoun HM, Dong W, Poulter NR. Blood pressure screening, management and control in England: results from the Health Survey for England 1994. *J Hypertens* 1998; **16**: 747–53.

20. Collins R, Peto R, MacMahon S, *et al.* Blood pressure, stroke, and coronary heat disease. Part 2, short-term reductions in blood pressure: overview of randomised drug trials in their epidemiological context. *Lancet* 1990; **335**: 827–39.
21. Materson BJ, Reda DJ, Cushman WC, *et al*, for the Department of Veterans Affairs Cooperative Study Group on Antihypertensive Agents. Single-drug therapy for hypertension in men. A comparison of six antihypertensive agents with placebo. *N Engl J Med* 1993; **328**: 914–21.
22. MacMahon S, Peto R, Cutler J, *et al.* Blood pressure, stroke, and coronary heart disease. Part 1, prolonged differences in blood pressure: prospective observational studies corrected for the regression dilution bias. *Lancet* 1990; **335**: 765–74.
23. United Kingdom Prospective Diabetes Study Group. Tight blood pressure control and risk of macrovascular and microvascular complications in type 2 diabetes. UKPDS 38. *BMJ* 1998; **317**; 703–13.
24. Hansson L, Zanchetti A, Carruthers SG, *et al.* for the HOT Study Group. Effects of intensive blood-pressure lowering and low-dose aspirin in patients with hypertension: principal results of the Hypertension Optimal Treatment (HOT) randomised trial. *Lancet* 1998; **351**: 1755–62.
25. Neaton JD, Grimm RH, Prineas RJ, *et al.* for the Treatment of Mild Hypertension Study Research Group. Treatment of Mild Hypertension Study. Final results. *JAMA* 1993; **270**: 713–24.
26. World Health Organization–International Society of Hypertension Blood Pressure Lowering Treatment Trialists' Collaboration. Protocol for prospective collaborative overviews of major randomized trials of blood-pressure-lowering treatments. *J Hypertens* 1998; **16**: 127–37.
27. Samuel O, Sakin P, Sybald B. *Counting on Quality: A Medical Audit Workbook.* London: Royal College of General Practitioners, 1993.
28. Royal College of Physicians. *Medical Audit: A First Report.* London: Royal College of Physicians, 1989.

Further Reading

Irvine, Irvine. *Making Sense of Audit*: Oxford: Radcliffe Medical Press.

Wayne C. *Clinical Audit.* London: Martin Dunitz, 1995.

chapter 9

Management of hypertension in subjects with other risk factors

As described in Chapter 6, cardiovascular risk factors tend to cluster in hypertensives, and furthermore the presence or absence of these risk factors greatly influences the outcome of hypertensives for any given level of BP. The implications are that these risk factors should be assessed in patients with hypertension (Chapter 7) and, assuming a tailored approach to management (Chapter 8), drug therapy may need to be modified in the light of the risk factor profile. Specific considerations for each of five major risk factors (obesity, diabetes, dyslipidaemia, insulin resistance and smoking) which frequently coexist among hypertensives are described in this chapter.

Obesity

Obesity and hypertension frequently coexist. In a recent survey of approximately 2000 hypertensive patients from 12 general practices in England, the majority had a BMI in excess of the ideal and 28% had a BMI above 30 kg/m^2 (obese) [1]. Increasing BMI appears to be causally related to higher levels of BP and, as shown in Figure 9.1, overweight is causally related to CHD incidence.

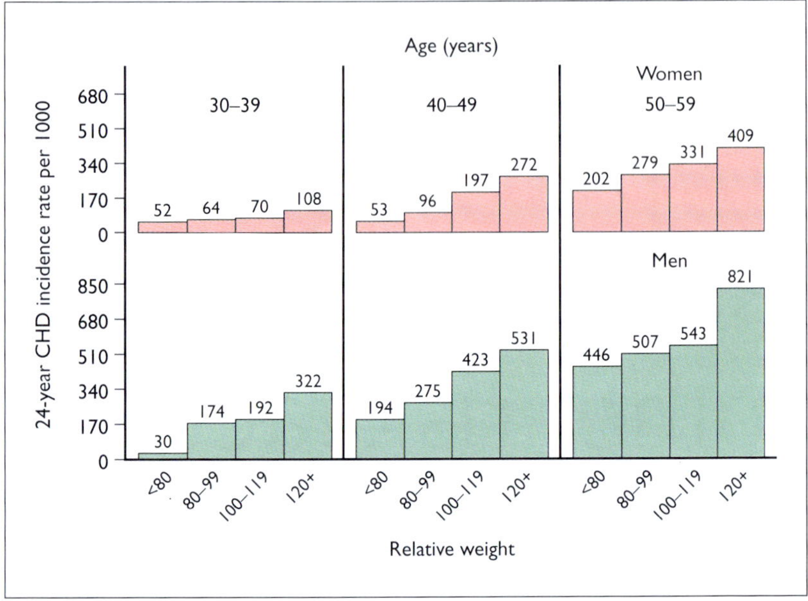

Figure 9.1. Relation of overweight to incidence of CHD.

Intervention trials of weight reduction have demonstrated that falls in both diastolic and systolic BP are associated with progressive degrees of weight loss in hypertensives and normotensives. On average, for every 1 kg of weight loss, a 2.5/1.5 mmHg reduction in BP is observed in hypertensives. Although many physicians are pessimistic about their ability to persuade their patients to lose weight, the potential benefit compared, for example, with that of β-blocker therapy has been clearly demonstrated (Fig. 9.2). The findings of this study also have important financial implications! All hypertensive patients who are overweight should be given systematic dietary advice to restrict calorie intake, and further weight loss may be facilitated by other measures outlined in Chapter 8. Few data are available to compare the relative efficacy of different pharmacological agents in obese hypertensive patients, but two factors are important when choosing the most appropriate drug for obese patients. First, varying degrees of obesity are associated with several concomitant adverse metabolic effects (Fig. 9.3). Second,

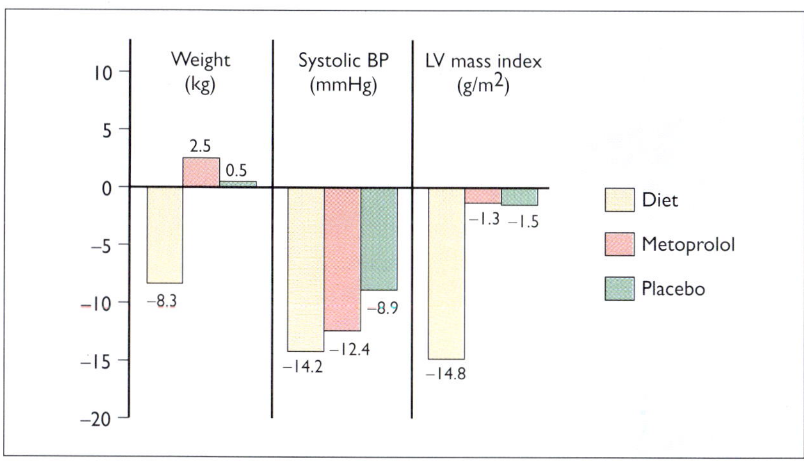

Figure 9.2. The effect of weight reduction compared with metoprolol, on BP and LV mass.

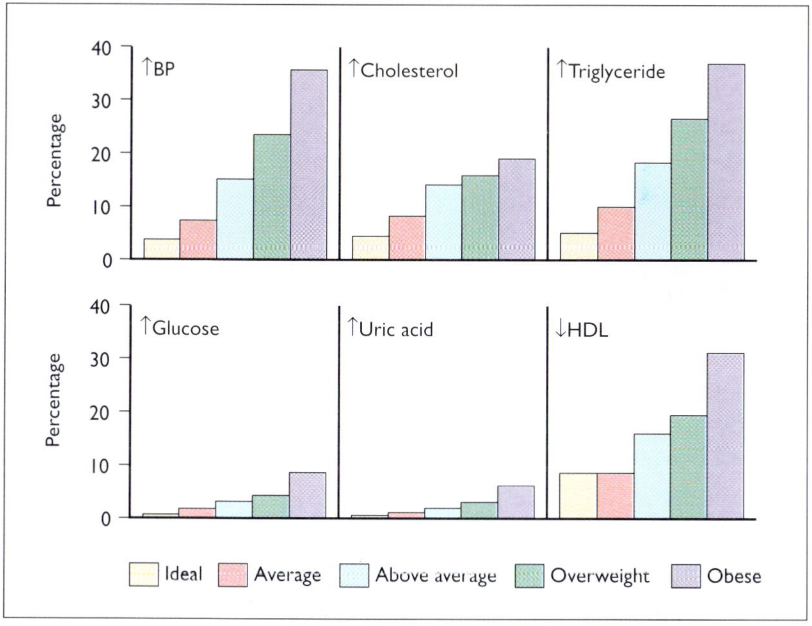

Figure 9.3. Association of degrees of obesity with concomitant adverse metabolic effects.

attempts to persuade patients to lose weight are hindered if β-blockers are prescribed, in part because they impair the ability of individuals to exercise.

In the absence of any trial evidence of BP-lowering therapy on this subgroup of patients, the optimal drug choice may be based on consideration of the need to exercise and of any dyslipidaemia and glucose intolerance, which so frequently coexist with obesity.

DIABETES

Approximately 50% of diabetic patients are hypertensive and, depending on the ethnic group (see Table 6.4), between 5 and 20% of hypertensive patients are diabetic. In addition, glucose intolerance is more common in hypertensives than among normotensives. Over 80% of diabetic subjects have non-insulin-dependent diabetes (NIDDM or type 2 diabetes), and hence are usually overweight and have a typical metabolic derangement, which includes a characteristic dyslipidaemia (as discussed in Chapter 6). As shown in Table 9.1, the risks associated with elevated BP are greatly enhanced by the coexistence of diabetes, which indicates that in this situation careful control of both conditions should be attempted. This suggestion has been confirmed by the findings of the United Kingdom Prospective Diabetes Study (UKPDS) [2] and Hypertension Optimal Treatment (HOT) [3] studies. The current consensus view, based on a 'best-estimate' rather than a trial approach, is that the BP threshold for drug treatment should be lowered in diabetics to 140 mmHg systolic and 90 mmHg diastolic, and, based on the HOT study [3], BPs should be lowered to <140 and <80 mmHg. These views are reinforced by the knowledge that reduction of BP, by whatever means, delays progression of vascular and renal damage in the diabetic patient [4].

Table 9.2 shows how the six major drug groups interact with those variables that should be considered when treating the diabetic. While loop diuretics produce less metabolic disturbance than thiazides, it

Table 9.1. Age-adjusted 10-year mortality by systolic BP and history of diabetes mellitus (Multiple Risk Factor Intervention Trial study)

Systolic BP quintile (mmHg)	Diabetic: Number	Diabetic: Number of deaths (rate per 1000)	Non-diabetic: Number	Non-diabetic: Number of deaths (rate per 1000)
<118	616	27 (40.0)	69 480	644 (10.3)
118–124	703	44 (54.8)	69 296	808 (12.8)
125–131	824	54 (52.3)	67 394	1018 (15.8)
132–141	1179	82 (57.3)	70 029	1456 (20.5)
≥142	1841	234 (104.0)	66 616	2774 (36.4)

seems clear from Table 9.2 that neither diuretics nor beta-blockers are expected to be optimal choices for the diabetic, particularly for those with NIDDM (in whom the metabolic derangement is so striking). This is supported by studies that have demonstrated the increased risk of developing diabetes associated with the use of diuretics and β-blockers (Fig. 9.4). The metabolic disturbances associated with NIDDM are less apparent in type I diabetes (IDDM) and hence the adverse effects of diuretics and β-blockers are perhaps less critical for patients with IDDM. However, despite these theoretical arguments, some of the limited trial evidence currently available [2,5] suggests that diuretics, and even β-blockers, may be suitable agents for managing hypertension in diabetic patients.

In the light of new evidence from several studies the picture has become, if anything, less clear. The Fosinopril versus Amlodipine Cardiovascular Events Randomized Trial (FACET) and Appropriate Blood Pressure Control in Diabetes (ABCD) studies suggested that ACE inhibitors should be preferred to dihydropyridine calcium antagonists. Indeed these data, along with other even less robust observational data,

Table 9.2. Special considerations for drug treatment of hypertension in diabetics

	Diuretic	β-blocker	α-blocker	ACE inhibitor	Calcium antagonist	AII antagonist
Nephropathy						
Serum K^+	↓*	–	–	↑	–	↑
Renal impairment	B	B	B	BB	B	B
Proteinuria	↓	↓	↓	↓↓	↓	↓↓
Neuropathy						
Impotence	AA	A	B	–	–	–
Orthostatic hypotension	A	A	AA†	–	–	–
Vascular						
PVD	?/A	A	–	–	–	?
Renal artery stenosis	–	–	–	AA	–	AA
CHD	?	BB	–	B	?/B	?/B
Metabolic						
HDL -C	–	↓	–/↑	–	–	–
LDL-C	↑	↑/↓	↓	–	–	–
Triglycerides	↑	↑	↓	–	–	–
Glucose	↑	↑	–	–	–	–
Insulin	↑	↑	↓	?/-	–	?/–
Obesity	–	A	–	–	–	–

Symbols: ↓reduction; ↑increase; – neutral or no data; ? uncertainties; A = adverse; B = beneficial.

*Except K^+-sparing agents where opposite effect may result.

†Short-acting agents only.

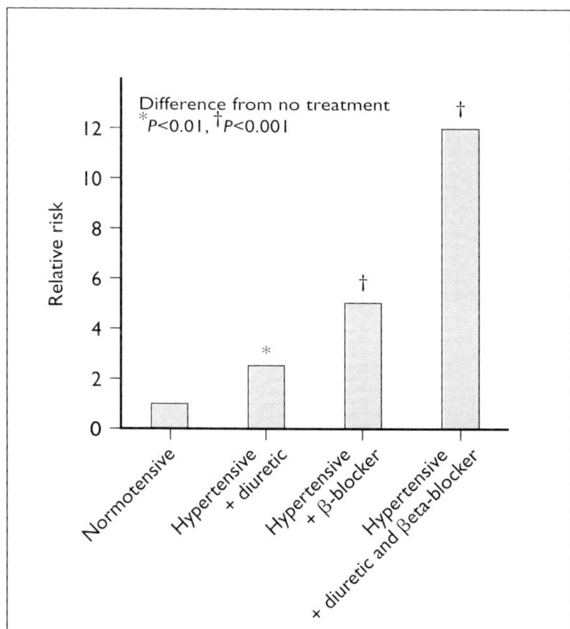

Figure 9.4. Increased risk of developing diabetes associated with the use of diuretics and β-blockers.

were misinterpreted to suggest that calcium antagonists were actually bad for diabetic patients [6]. To conflict with this message, the diabetic subgroup in the SYST-EUR trial [7] showed huge reductions on all cardiovascular events associated with the use of nitrendipine (Table 9.3)

The UKPDS trial results have also been published recently [2]. This trial, which had been carried out over 20 years, did provide some answers, but also raised more controversy – particularly in the hypertension management part of the trial, which was a late add-on feature to the main study. The idea was to determine whether tight BP control with either atenolol or captopril had a specific advantage in preventing complications in type 2 diabetics, compared with less tight control.

About one-third of the diabetic patients were randomized and treated to bring BP down to <180/<105 mmHg without using an ACE inhibitor or a β-blocker (less tight control). The remainder were randomized, less effectively than might have been hoped, into two

Table 9.3. The SYST-EUR trial: benefits of antihypertensive treatment in diabetic patients*

	End points/1000 patient-years (no. of events)		Percentage	
	Placebo (*n* = 240)	Active treatment (*n* = 252)	Benefit of treatment (95% CI)	P value
Mortality				
Overall	45.1 (26)	26.4 (16)	41 (–9 to 69)	0.09
Cardiovascular causes	27.8 (16)	8.3 (5)	70 (19 to 89)	0.01
Fatal and nonfatal end points				
All cardiovascular events	57.6 (31)	22.0 (13)	62 (19 to 80)	0.002
Stroke	26.6 (15)	8.3 (5)	69 (14 to 89)	0.02
Cardiac events	27.1 (15)	11.7 (7)	57 (–6 to 82)	0.06

*The benefit is expressed as the percent reduction in the event rate for the active treatment group; negative numbers indicate increases in the event rate; CI denotes confidence interval.

groups and treated to bring BP down to <150/<85 mmHg either by using captopril 25 mg twice daily, increasing to 50 mg twice daily, or by using atenolol 50 mg once a day, increasing to 100 mg once daily, along with a series of stipulated add-on drugs as required for either group (tight control). The three groups achieved mean BPs of 154/87 mmHg, 144/83 mmHg and 143/81 mmHg, respectively.

The pivotal message to arise from this part of the UKPDS trial is that tight BP control in hypertensive patients with type 2 diabetes achieves clinically important reduction in the risk of deaths related to diabetes, complications related to diabetes, progression of retinopathy and deterioration in visual acuity, compared with a less tight control (Table 9.4). Furthermore, the benefits associated with tight BP control are greater than those associated with intensive versus less intensive glucose control!

As to whether captopril or atenolol was more effective, no differences were detected, but the trial was grossly underpowered to evaluate this. In practice, the study has been widely misinterpreted to mean that the two drugs are equally effective.

A subgroup analysis of the diabetics included in the HOT trial has reinforced the message that to lower BP aggressively is very important in these patients [3]. The HOT trial was designed to establish whether the incremental benefits of lowering BP to ≤90, ≤85 or ≤80 mmHg

Table 9.4. The impact of tight BP control in UKPDS[2]

Clinical end point	Absolute risk (events per 1000 patient years) Tight control	Less tight control	P value	Relative risk for tight control (95% CI)
Any diabetes-related end point	50.9	67.4	0.0046	0.76 (0.62–0.92)
Deaths related to diabetes	13.7	20.3	0.019	0.68 (0.49–0.94)
All cause mortality	22.4	27.2	0.17	0.82 (0.63–1.08)
Myocardial infarction	18.6	23.5	0.13	0.79 (0.59–1.07)
Stroke	6.5	11.6	0.013	0.56 (0.35–0.89)
Peripheral vascular disease	1.4	2.7	0.17	0.51 (0.19–1.37)
Microvascular disease	12.0	19.2	0.0092	0.63 (0.44–0.89)

were apparent in terms of preventing cardiovascular events. In the diabetic patients it was clear that the lower the BP, the fewer the cardiovascular endpoints. However, it must be stressed that to achieve a lowering of diastolic BP to <90 mmHg most patients needed at least two drugs.

In the diabetic subgroup of the Captopril Prevention Project (CAPPP) trial [8], in which patients were randomized to either a captopril-based regimen or 'usual' therapy (usually β-blocker based), those who received an ACE inhibitor tended to do better in terms of all cardiovascular events except stroke. However, this trial had several serious shortcomings – not least the inadequate (usually once daily) dosing with captopril.

Hence, despite these subgroup analyses, one of the most important questions regarding therapy for these hypertensive diabetic patients remains whether particular benefits are conferred by any individual class of antihypertensive agent over and above those produced by BP lowering, particularly with respect to major cardiovascular events in this high-risk group. Currently, several studies are addressing this important issue.

Meanwhile, one study has shown that deterioration in renal function is significantly reduced in patients with IDDM – supposedly independently of any BP-lowering effect – by the use of ACE inhibitors [9]. This resulted in the recommendation of the preferential use of ACE inhibitors for patients with IDDM and proteinuria. However, the key message in diabetic hypertensives appears to be – bring the BP down!

Pending long-awaited robust trial evidence, and given the variable effects on renal and sexual function, dyslipidaemia and urinary microalbuminuria, better choices for patients with hypertension and diabetes might be AII antagonists, calcium antagonists or α-blockers, except following myocardial infarction, in which case β-blockers in combination with a lipid-lowering agent remain the preferred drug group. In reality, to achieve a sufficient lowering of BP, all the major drug classes are often needed in combinations.

DYSLIPIDAEMIA

Elevated BP is usually associated with an abnormal serum lipid profile [1]. Over 85% of hypertensive patients in a study from 12 English general practices had a total cholesterol level above the ideal (>5.2 mmol/l) (Table 9.5), about 65% had levels above 6.0 mmol/l (which doubles the risk of a CHD event), and the mean level was approximately 6.5 mmol/l. There is also evidence that a significant proportion of hypertensive patients have other lipid abnormalities (low HDL cholesterol and high triglycerides) that are associated with the insulin-resistance syndrome (see chapter 6). Since the principal aim of treating hypertension in a westernized population is to prevent heart attacks and strokes, it seems logical that coexisting cardiovascular risk factors, including abnormal lipid profiles, should be an integral part of hypertension management.

All recent national and international guidelines recommend measurement of lipid profiles in hypertensives and advocate appropriate intervention as required. These recommendations are based on data such as those shown in Figure 6.5, which clearly demonstrate that having a below-average serum cholesterol (<6.5 mmol/l) has a greater impact on the prognosis for hypertensives than does antihypertensive therapy [10]. Further evidence of the independent effect of increasing levels of lipids among hypertensives is shown in Table 6.2 [11]. A clear

Table 9.5. Distribution of cholesterol levels in 1948 hypertensive patients from 12 general practices in England

Cholesterol level (mmol/l)	Male (%)	Female (%)
<5.2	17.1	10.2
5.2–<6.5	47.6	34.0
6.5–<7.8	26.7	36.8
≥7.8	8.7	19.0

dose–response effect of serum cholesterol on death from CHD is apparent among smokers and non-smokers irrespective of BP level.

Support for intervention in patients who have coexistent abnormal lipids and hypertension (if one is present, the other usually is) comes from the Gothenburg Primary Prevention Study (Fig. 9.5) [12], which shows that coronary risk is not greatly reduced with BP reduction if serum cholesterol rises (e.g. the green group). However, among those patients in whom both BP and serum cholesterol were reduced, large reductions in coronary risk were achieved. The benefit of lowering BP and cholesterol is undergoing further evaluation in two large-scale trials [13,14].

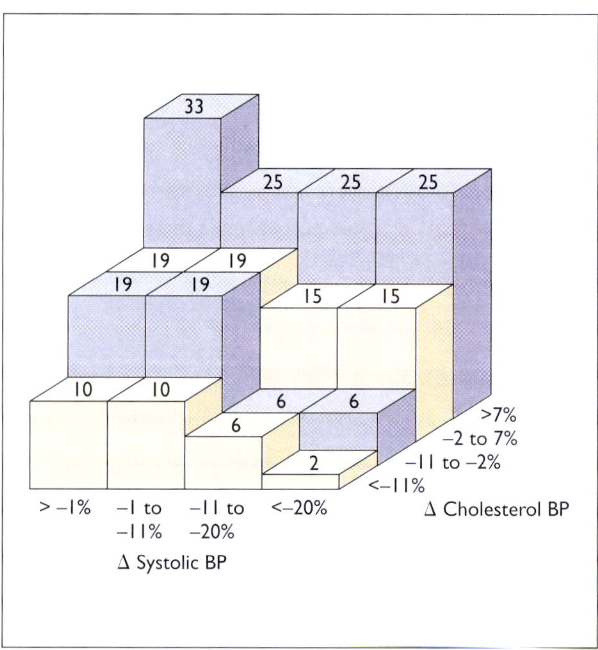

Figure 9.5. Impact on coronary risk by changes in systolic BP and cholesterol.

The cornerstone of managing the hyperlipidaemic hypertensive patient is dietary and lifestyle advice. In addition to the standard advice for hypertensives (Chapter 8), these patients require advice as to how to reduce saturated fat and cholesterol intake, reduce total calories (when overweight) and increase exercise output.

Doctors have become nihilistic about their ability to influence blood lipid profiles. However, a recent editorial review of the benefit of diets said:

> *Despite scepticism about difficulties in modifying plasma cholesterol concentrations with diet, a recent review of 420 dietary observations from 141 groups of subjects showed clearly that a reduction of 10% in the proportion of energy derived from saturated fatty acids would be associated with a plasma cholesterol concentration 0.5 mmol/l lower. These data suggest that this would yield a substantial reduction in death from CHD.*

The choice of antihypertensive drugs in the dyslipidaemic patient is unclear. Conventional doses of diuretics and β-blockers have small adverse effects on the serum lipid profile (Table 9.7). Although undoubtedly small, these effects may be biologically important and confer a significant and important increase in the risk of CHD in patients who are already at risk because of their higher levels of BP and abnormal lipid profiles. The α-blockers have a favourable effect on serum lipids, whereas ACE inhibitors and calcium antagonists have a neutral effect, as demonstrated in the Treatment of Mild Hypertension Study (TOMHS) study (Fig. 9.6). Also, AII antagonists have no adverse effects on lipid profiles. Recommendations have been made based on randomized trial evidence [15] that dictates that almost all patients who have angina or who suffer a myocardial infarction should receive lipid-lowering therapy. In addition, among those patients who do not have established vascular disease, best evidence suggests that those at highest risk should receive lipid lowering with statin drugs [16]. Methods of identifying those at high risk are discussed below (see Chapter 8, 'Absolute risk scores').

Table 9.7. Effects of diuretics and β-blockers on serum lipids

	Percentage change			
	Total cholesterol	HDL	LDL	Triglyceride
Diuretic	+4	+10	0	+9
β-blockers				
non-selective	0	0	–7	+29
selective	0	0	–7	+18
plus ISA	0	0	–2	+13

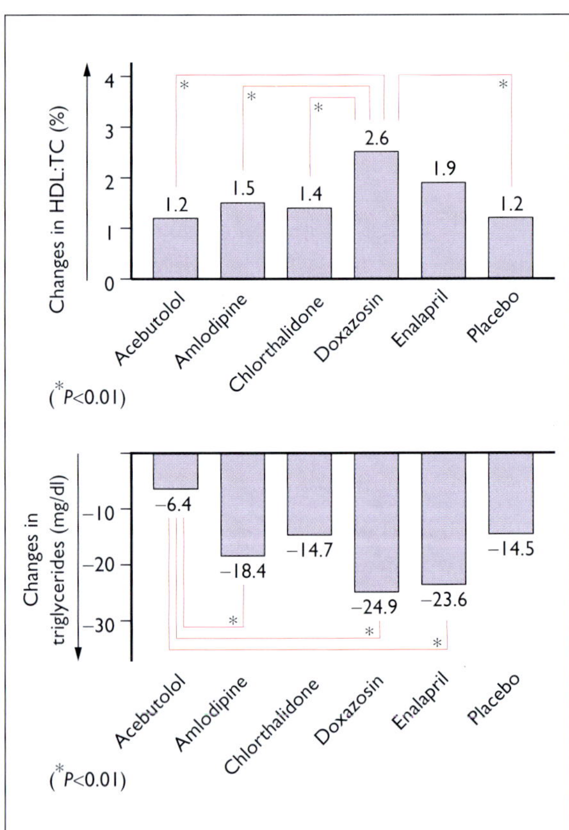

Figure 9.6. Study demonstrating the effects on serum lipids of various antihypertensive agents [14].

INSULIN RESISTANCE

The principal therapeutic implication of insulin resistance is that it serves to emphasize that non-pharmacological approaches, and particularly weight loss and increased exercise, form the cornerstone of the management of diabetes, hypertension and obesity.

The different impact of various drugs on insulin resistance as measured by euglycaemic clamp techniques, as described in Chapter 6, is shown in Figure 9.7. As might be predicted from the effects on lipid subfractions, the most beneficial effects are observed in association with

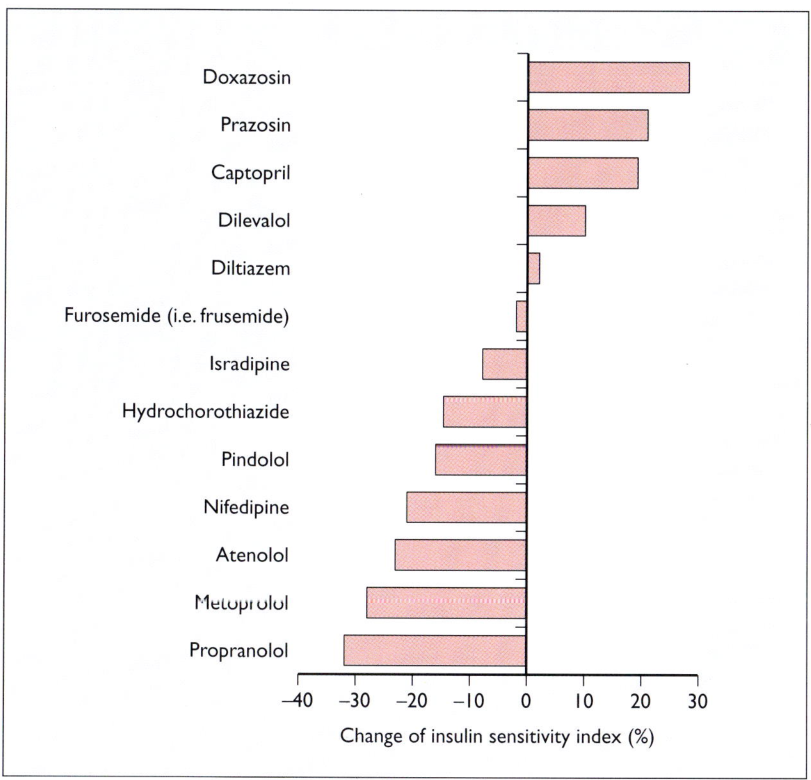

Figure 9.7. The different impact of various drugs on insulin resistance as measured by euglycaemic clamp techniques.

the use of α-blockers and the most adverse effects with β-blockers. However, no randomized trial evidence is as yet available to compare the efficacy of these two drug groups in terms of cardiovascular disease prevention among insulin-resistant patients.

Assuming insulin resistance contributes to hyperglycemia in patients with type 2 diabetes, improving insulin sensitivity will undoubtedly improve glycemic control. The discovery of a new class of 'insulin sensitizers', the peroxisome proliferator activated receptor agonists (PPAR γ), also known as the thiazolidinediones, is an exciting development.

The PPAR γ is a ligand-activated nuclear receptor which is the primary molecular target for the thiazolidinedione class of insulin-sensitizing agents. It is known that the binding of these compounds to PPAR γ is highly correlated with their anti-diabetic insulin-sensitizing potency. The consequence of this activation *in vivo* is to reduce insulin resistance. Importantly, skeletal muscle and adipose tissue, glucose transport and glucose transporters are increased. Also, in the liver there is an enhanced suppression of hepatic glucose output in response to insulin 11.

Clinical studies have shown that activation of PPAR γ via thiazolidinediones (for example rosiglitazone) [12] translates into a durable anti-hyperglycaemic effect in patients with type 2 diabetes. Existing pharmacological treatments for type 2 diabetes all have drawbacks. The sulfonylurea drugs act by stimulating secretion of insulin from functioning pancreatic beta cells. The main drawback of the group is the induction hyper-insulinaemia, which can lead to hypoglycaemia and weight gain. At best, only 60–70% of patients will reach glycaemic targets with sulphonylurea therapy. The biguanides (for example metformin) lower blood glucose mainly by inhibiting hepatic glucose production. There may be reluctance to take this drug because it causes some gastro-intestinal symptoms leading to poor compliance. The alpha glucosidase inhibitors (for example acarbose) reduce post-prandial glucose peaks by retarding the absorption of glucose from the intestines. The common side effects are flatulence, diarrhoea and abdominal bloating.

The management of type 2 diabetes requires a holistic approach to achieve good glycemic control. UKPDS has demonstrated the value of achieving tight BP control with clinically important reductions in the risk of complications and deaths related to diabetes 13. It is also critically important to manage lipid abnormalities appropriately. The need for new and effective medications that target the underlying cause of type 2 diabetes insulin resistance has become more achievable with the advent of an effective new class of agents known as glitazones or thiazolidinediones which will have the potential for preventing the progression of type 2 diabetes.

SMOKING

The prevalence of smoking is declining in many westernized societies, although in eastern Europe and many developing countries smoking rates are increasing. In the UK, about 29% of male and 27% of female adults smoke cigarettes, but it is worrying that the prevalence of smoking in men and women aged 16–24 is 36% and 37%, respectively, and is increasing [17]. Furthermore, increasing numbers of young women are taking up smoking. In a recent survey of hypertensives from 12 general practices in England, 20% of hypertensive patients smoked [1]. This is of particular importance, since smoking markedly increases the risk of developing CHD and stroke associated with hypertension.

Some studies show that smokers have lower levels of BP than non-smokers, even after correcting the data for differences in body weight (smokers also tend to be thinner). This may be misleading, however, because BP is invariably taken when the patient is not smoking, whereas BP increases acutely during smoking through a number of mechanisms, including sympathetic stimulation. Continuous BP monitoring in heavy smokers suggests that BP levels are increased for much of the day (i.e. during smoking), and paired home BP recordings in a large national survey in the UK confirm higher BP levels among heavy-smoking males. In keeping with these observations is that more severe forms of hypertension, including accelerated phase or malignant hypertension, are much more likely to occur in the hypertensive patient who smokes.

Figure 9.8 shows the impact of smoking on the risk of developing a myocardial infarction and a stroke among those treated in the Medical Research Council hypertension trial. These data confirm that the most important advice to give to the hypertensive smoker is to stop smoking, since any benefits from cessation of smoking are likely to be greater than those conferred by antihypertensive drugs.

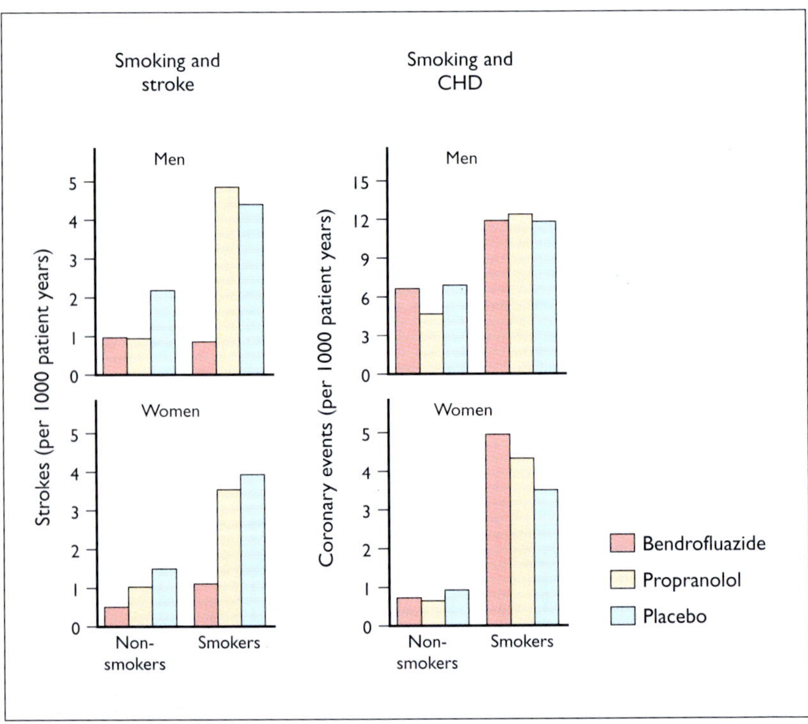

Figure 9.8. The impact of smoking on the risk of developing a myocardial infarction and a stroke among those treated in the Medical Research Council hypertension trial.

There is evidence (bearing in mind reservations about post-hoc subgroup analyses) from at least one trial that therapeutic responses to β-blockers are reduced in the smoking hypertensive and hence, based on the trial evidence available to date, diuretics may be preferable to β-blockers in patients who smoke. From a mechanistic point of view, as yet unsupported by any trial evidence, α-blockers or calcium antagonists may be more effective by preventing nicotine-induced vasospasm (Fig. 9.9).

Heavy smokers often suffer from chronic bronchitis and/or COPD. In this situation, as in asthma, β-blockers are unsuitable because of their tendency to cause bronchospasm. These patients are also prone to coughing and it can often be difficult to evaluate whether cough associated with the use of ACE inhibitors results from the drug or the underlying respiratory condition.

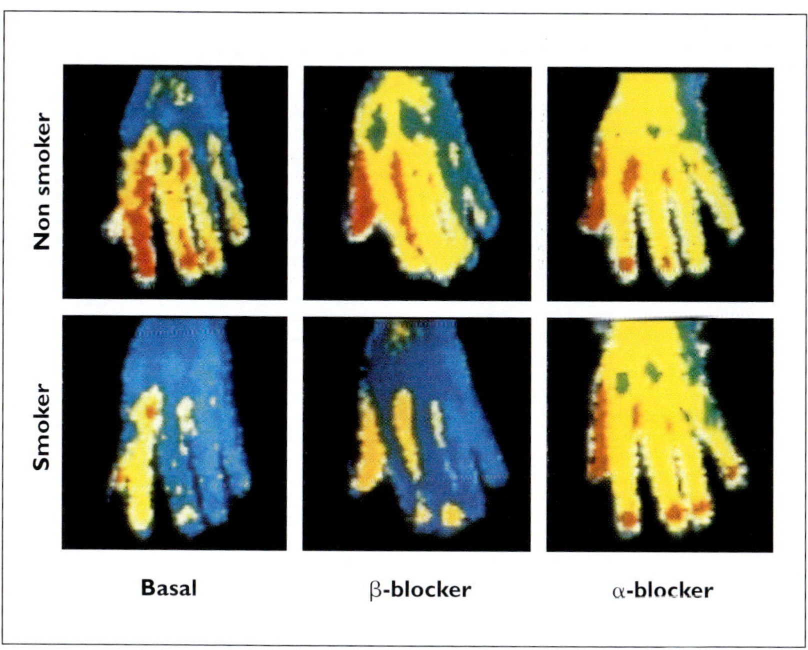

Figure 9.9. Prevention of nicotine-induced peripheral vasoconstriction by an α-blocker, as indicated by skin temperature.

Chapter Summary

- Cardiovascular risk factors tend to cluster in hypertensive patients.
- The presence or absence of these risk factors greatly influences the outcome of hypertensives at any given level of BP. Risk factors should be assessed in all patients with hypertension.
- Assuming a tailored approach to the management, drug therapy may need to be modified in the light of the overall risk profile.
- Specific consideration needs to be given to obesity, diabetes, dyslipidaemia, insulin resistance, LVH and smoking.
- The optimal management of dyslipidaemia for patients with hypertension is best achieved by basing the intervention upon absolute risk of cardiovascular disease after taking into account levels of other risk factors.
- The use of aspirin for patients with hypertension should be dependent on careful consideration of several specified criteria, for example age and BP control.

References

1. Poulter NR, Zographos D, Mattin R, Sever PS, Thom S McG. Concomitant risk factors in hypertensives: A survey of risk factors for cardiovascular disease amongst hypertensives in English general practices. *Blood Pressure* 1996; **5**(4): 209–15.
2. United Kingdom Prospective Diabetes Study Group. Tight blood pressure control and risk of macrovascular and microvascular complications in type 2 diabetes. UKPDS 38. *Br Med J* 1998; **317**: 703–13.
3. Hansson L, Zanchetti A, Carruthers SG, *et al.* for the HOT Study Group. Effects of intensive blood-pressure lowering and low-dose aspirin in patients with hypertension: principal results of the Hypertension Optimal Treatment (HOT) randomised trial. *Lancet* 1998; **351**: 1755–62.

4. Parving HH. Impact of blood pressure and antihypertensive treatment on incipient and overt nephropathy, retinopathy, and endothelial permeability in diabetes mellitus. *Diabetes Care* 1991; **14**: 260–9.
5. SHEP Cooperative Research Group. Prevention of stroke by antihypertensive drug treatment in older persons with isolated systolic hypertension. Final results of the Systolic Hypertension in the Elderly Program (SHEP). *JAMA* 1991; **265**: 3255–64.
6. Poulter NR. Calcium antagonists and the diabetic patient: a response to recent controversies. *Am J Cardiol* 1998; **82**; 40R–41R.
7. Tuomilehto J, Rastenyte D, Birkenhager WH, *et al.* Effects of calcium-channel blockade in older patients with diabetes and systolic hypertension. Syst Eur Investigators. *N Engl J Med* 1999; **340**: 677–84.
8. Hansson L, Lindholm LH, Niskanen L, *et al.* Effect of angiotensin-converting enzyme inhibition compared with conventional therapy on cardiovascular morbidity and mortality in hypertension: the Captopril Prevention Project (CAPPP). *Lancet* 1999; **353**: 611–5.
9. Lewis EJ, Hunsicker LG, Bain RP, Rohde RD, for the Collaborative Study Group. The effect of angiotensin-converting-enzyme inhibition on diabetic nephropathy. *N Engl J Med* 1993; **329**: 1456–62.
10. Biochemical characteristics, their changes due to antihypertensive treatment, and their prognostic value. In: Miall WE, Greenberg G, eds. *Mild Hypertension – Is There Pressure to Treat?* Cambridge: Cambridge University Press, 1987: 145–52.
11. Stamler J. Established major coronary risk factors. In: Marmot M, Elliott P, eds. *Coronary Heart Disease Epidemiology: From Aetiology to Public Health.* Oxford: Oxford University Press, 1992; 35–66.
12. Samuelson O Wilhelmson L, Andersson OK, *et al.* Cardiovascular morbidity in relation to changes in blood pressure and serum cholesterol level in treated hypertension. *JAMA* 1987; **258**: 1768–76.
13. Davis BR, Cutler JA, Gordon DJ, *et al.* Rationale and design for the Antihypertensive and Lipid Lowering Treatment to prevent Heart Attack Trial (ALLHAT). *Am J Hypertens* 1996; **9**: 342–60.
14. Neaton JD, Grimm RH, Prineas RJ *et al.* Treatment of mild hypertension study. *J Am Med Assoc* 1993; **270**: 713–24
15. Dahlof B, Sever PS, Poulter NR, Wedel H. On behalf of the ASCOT Steering Committee. International Society of Hypertension. *J Hypertens* 1998; **16** (Suppl. 2): S212.

16. Wood D, Durrington P, Poulter N, McInnes G, Rees A, Wray R for the British Cardiac Society, British Hyperlipidaemia Association, British Hypertension Society, and British Diabetic Association. Joint British recommendations on prevention of coronary heart disease in clinical practice. *Heart* 1998; **80**: S1–S29.
17. Ramsay LE, Johnston GD, MacGregor GA, *et al.* Guidelines for Management of Hypertension: Report of the third working party of the British Hypertension Society. *J Hum Hypertens* 1999; **13**(9): 569–92.
18. Colhoun HM, Prescott-Clarke P. *The Health Survey for England 1994.* London: HMSO; 1996.

chapter 10

Special situations

Chapter 1 describes the treatment of hypertension by non-pharmacological and pharmacological means. This chapter deals with several additional circumstances that warrant specific mention (Table 10.1).

Table 10.1. Special situations in hypertensive patient management

The elderly		Conn's syndrome
Pregnancy	2° hypertension	Phaeochromocytoma
Children		Renal artery stenosis
Urgencies/emergencies	Resistant hypertension	
Heart failure	Alcohol & drug-induced hypertension	
Renal failure	Compliance	

The Elderly

BP rises with age in westernized populations – as discussed in Chapter 3. This is a pathological accompaniment to the ageing process and reflects structural changes in the vasculature that occur throughout life. These changes may develop from continuous exposure to a diet that contains quantities of salt and fat far in excess of our metabolic requirements, to smoking or to hypertension itself. Structural changes in the large arteries lead to increased stiffness of the vasculature, augmentation of systolic BP and a fall in diastolic pressure – isolated systolic hypertension [1]. This pattern of isolated systolic hypertension with a wide pulse pressure is frequently encountered in the elderly (Fig. 10.1) and in itself is associated with increased morbidity and mortality (Fig. 10.2 and see Chapter 5) [2].

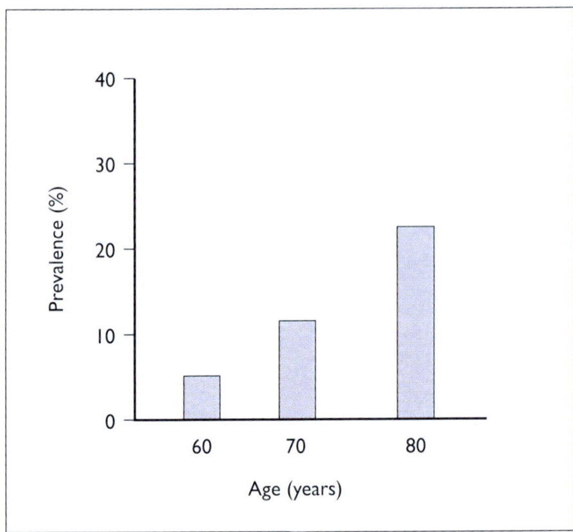

Figure 10.1. Prevalence of isolated systolic hypertension increasing with age.

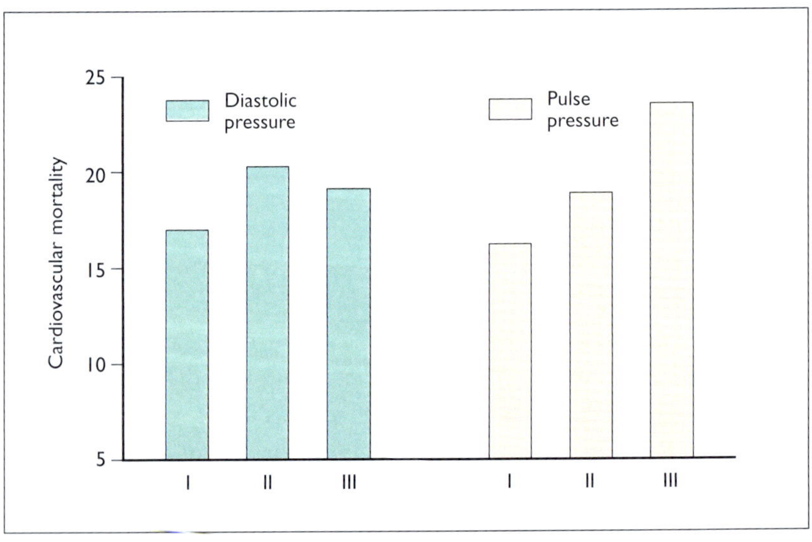

Figure 10.2. Mortality by tertiles of BP in patients with heart failure indicating the dominant influence of widening pulse pressure [2].

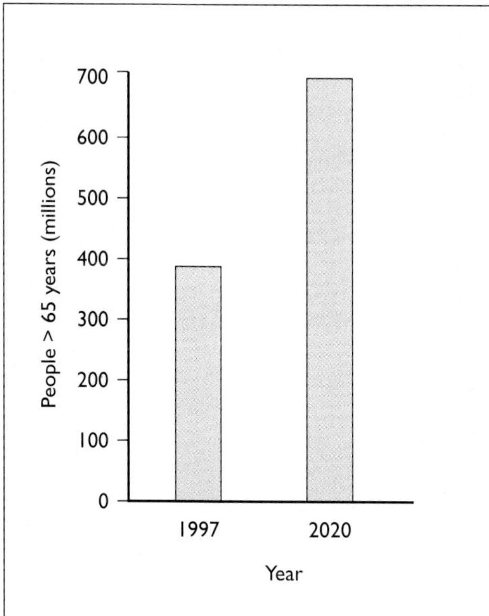

Figure 10.3. Numbers of the world population over 65 years; now and projection for 2020 [3].

In affluent societies, life expectancy is increasing (Fig. 10.3). The population is ageing such that for every baby born in a westernized country there are 10 people aged 65 years or over. By the year 2020 there will be 15 such elderly people for each newborn [3].

Drug treatment for systolic hypertension in the elderly

Large numbers of people over 60 years of age have levels of BP that warrant treatment (Fig. 10.4), and the elderly are at increased risk of cardiovascular events related to hypertension. On these grounds we might consider lowering the threshold at which we define their hypertension and introduce therapy, but this would imply treating the majority of elderly people. Faced with this awesome prospect, most specialist guidelines offer the pragmatic advice:

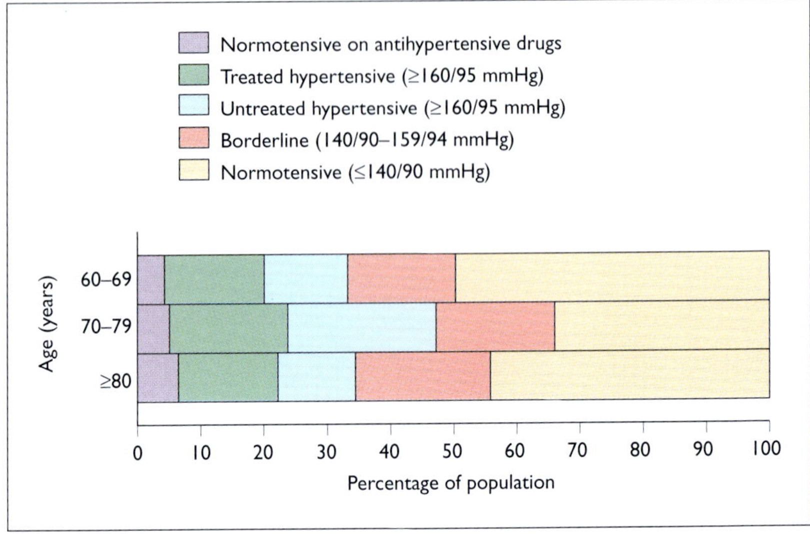

Figure 10.4. Categories of hypertensive patients aged 60 years and over in Britain.

- that BP thresholds for initiating treatment remain the same in the elderly as for younger patients
- that target BP for older patients remains the same as for younger patients.

These targets may necessarily be adjusted in the face of very high starting pressures.

Several trials in the elderly (see Chapter 12) show marked benefit from drug treatments, at least up to the age of 80 years (once started there is no sound reason to stop treatment on a patient's 80th birthday). Trials in the 'elderly elderly' are currently under way for those over 80 years of age, and meanwhile it is reasonable to base treatment decisions on biological rather than chronological age. It is also important to dispel the myth that the elderly tolerate medication less well. Equally, the non-pharmacological measures of salt restriction, weight reduction and increased physical activity may be helpful manoeuvres in this group of patients (Fig. 10.5) [4]. Significant salt restriction is difficult to achieve as at least 75% of our customary dietary salt intake is added to food in the course of processing by the food industry. However, the BP of the elderly is particularly sensitive to salt.

Most of the hypertension treatment trials have systematically excluded patients with other complicating conditions such as angina, COPD, gout, etc. With increasing age multiple concurrent problems accumulate. Table 10.2 provides suggestions for the optimal drugs for patients with various coexistent problems. Atherosclerotic renovascular disease may cause or complicate hypertension more frequently in the elderly patient who typically would be a biologically old, male smoker with claudication. ACE inhibitors and angiotensin receptor blockers are relatively contraindicated in this setting because of the attendant risk of renal impairment (Fig. 10.6).

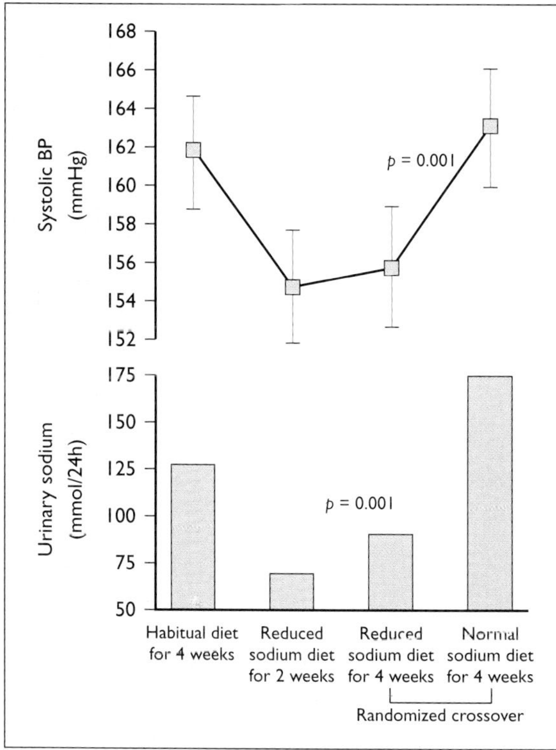

Figure 10.5. An elderly untreated group (systolic BP range 123–205 mmHg) completed a 2-month randomised crossover of salt restriction with slow sodium and placebo to give salt intake of either 10g or 5g. Urinary sodium was measured to reflect the dietary changes. A reduction in sodium intake of 83 mmol/day was associated with a 7.2/3.2 mmHg BP reduction. Hypertensives and nomotensives responded similarly. (After Cappuccio [4]).

Based on evidence from the Systolic Hypertension in the Elderly Program (SHEP) and SYST-EUR trials, thiazides or dihydropyridine calcium antagonists are preferred drug treatments in isolated systolic hypertension.

Table 10.2. Coexisting disease in the elderly hypertensive: implications for drug therapy

Coexisting disease	Drug group					
	Diuretic	β-blocker	Calcium antagonist enzyme	ACE inhibitor	α-blocker antagonist	AII
None	++	+	–	+	+	+
CCF	++	–	0/–*	++	?	+(+)
Angina	–	++	++	0	0	0
COPD	+	–	+	–	+	+
PVD	–	–	++	–	++	–
Gout	–	+	+	+	+	+
DM/IGT	–	–	+	++	++	+
BPH	–	+	0	+	++	+
ED	–	–	?	?	++	?

++ Optimal drug; + possible alternative; 0 less suitable;
– caution/contraindicated; ? uncertain, potentially.
*Depending on type of calcuim antagonist.

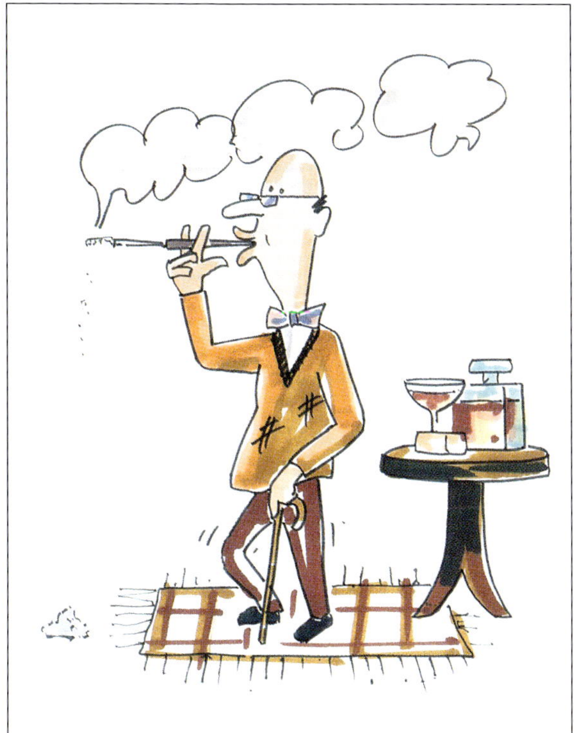

Figure 10.6. The older male smoking claudicant in whom ACE inhibitors and AII antagonists are relatively contraindicated.

Pregnancy, the pill, and hormone replacement therapy

Hypertension complicates up to 10% of pregnancies. In a mild form, whether chronic or induced by the pregnancy, it poses little risk to the mother or fetus, but pre-eclampsia and eclampsia, which generally occur with more severe hypertension, are major causes of serious fetal and maternal problems, including death.

Pre-eclampsia is largely a disorder of first pregnancies in which the incidence is between 4 and 5% [5]. It is a much less frequent problem in subsequent pregnancies, unless the mother changes partner. The risks to the mother include eclamptic convulsions, cerebral haemorrhage, pulmonary oedema, renal and hepatic failure, disseminated intravascular coagulation and death. The risks to the fetus result from placental insufficiency (effectively oxygen and nutrient starvation), intrauterine growth retardation, asphyxia and abruptio placentae.

The normal haemodynamic changes of pregnancy include a fall in BP towards the end of the first trimester, which follows a reduction in peripheral vascular resistance. The absence of this fall is found in those women with chronic hypertension or it may be predictive of an imminent hypertensive disorder. Subsequently, BP rises towards (or even transiently above) nonpregnant levels at term. In patients with pre-eclampsia or eclampsia, this BP rise is usually exaggerated and occurs earlier in the pregnancy, although raised BP levels are not a necessary part of this syndrome. Four categories of hypertension associated with pregnancy are observed (Table 10.3).

Treatment of raised BP in pre-eclampsia is primarily directed at prevention of maternal complications. Only delivery of the baby corrects established eclampsia. In severe cases, there is a difficult balance to strike between the safety of the mother and buying more time *in utero* for fetal development. In rare cases, pre-eclampsia may progress to maternal convulsions (eclampsia) in the first day or two immediately post delivery. Important warning signs indicative of pre-eclampsia are given in Table 10.4.

Most physicians and obstetricians take a BP threshold of ≥140/90 mmHg for starting drug treatment; certainly treatment is indicated at BP ≥160/100 mmHg. Korotkoff phase V is the accepted point for measurement of diastolic pressure. Perhaps even more important than the given level of BP is the increment in pressure with progression of the pregnancy – for instance, a woman whose BP rises to a systolic 140 mmHg at 30 weeks from 100 mmHg at booking may well be in trouble.

Methyldopa is the antihypertensive agent that has been most extensively evaluated in pregnancy [6]. β-blockers (atenolol and metoprolol) appear reasonably safe and effective, but only in the latter part of pregnancy because fetal growth retardation has been identified in the offspring of mothers treated with atenolol in the first trimester. Both

Table 10.3. Hypertensive disorders associated with pregnancy

■ Chronic hypertension	Known disorder before pregnancy or rise in BP to >140/90 mmHg before 20 weeks
■ Pre-eclampsia	Rise in BP of >15 mmHg diastolic or >30 mmHg systolic from early pregnancy
■ Pre-eclampsia superimposed on chronic hypertension	
■ Transient/late gestational hypertension	Rise in blood pressure as for pre-eclampsia, without proteinuria; resolves within post-partum weeks

Table 10.4. Symptoms and signs of pre-eclampsia

- Headache
- Epigastric discomfort
- Hepatic tenderness
- Advancing proteinuria
- Marked oedema
- Brisk reflexes with clonus
- Rising BP (loss of nocturnal BP dip)
- Reduced fetal activity

ACE inhibitors and angiotensin II-receptor blockers should be avoided because of serious risk to the fetus, particularly in the second and third trimesters of pregnancy. Generally, these agents should not be used for hypertension control in fertile young women in the first instance. If taken before pregnancy and at the time of conception, diuretics and, perhaps, calcium antagonists might reasonably be continued – although there is little published data to support the use of calcium antagonists in this situation. For the reasons stated above, many physicians advocate switching to methyldopa when pregnancy is confirmed. Large trials have not shown any benefit from prophylactic low-dose aspirin or supplemental calcium in the prevention of pre-eclampsia.

Too frequently young women with established chronic hypertension are warned against pregnancy. Chronic essential hypertension is not a contraindication to pregnancy – in most cases the BP follows the normal profile of changes through pregnancy, the hypertension is mild and the pregnancy uncomplicated. Pre-existing therapy can often be withdrawn early on. The development of pre-eclampsia may be more likely, but is still unusual. The situation warrants careful antenatal monitoring – not proscription. However, women with unrecognized secondary causes of hypertension may do badly in pregnancy.

In acute hypertension, or a hypertensive pre-eclamptic crisis, the rate of rise of BP is probably more critical than the absolute level – eclamptic convulsions may occur at relatively low levels of BP and 'hypertension' is not an absolute component of the pre-eclamptic syndrome. Urgent measures need to be taken to deliver the baby; meanwhile parenteral hydralazine or labetalol can be administered. Oral nifedipine retard may be effective relatively quickly, although the side effect of headache may confuse the clinical picture. There is no place for the use of sublingual and/or capsular nifedipine here or in any other medical setting, as it may have an extremely brisk effect in causing a precipitous fall in BP. Such a rapid reduction in the already critical perfusion of the brain, heart and placenta may have catastrophic consequences – infarction of these organs. If magnesium sulphate is being used for seizure prophylaxis, the use of calcium antagonists may dangerously augment hypotension.

Transient or late-gestational hypertension predicts the development of essential hypertension. The association of pre-eclampsia with future hypertension is less clear, although some data do suggest a positive link. It does appear that a history of pre-eclampsia may predict a hypertensive response to the combined oral contraceptive (OC) pill and also thrombotic complications of the pill.

The pill

On average, the combined OC pill produces a small rise in BP of about 5/3 mmHg. In most women, BP remains within the normal range, but a few become clearly hypertensive. The BP response is directly related to the oestrogen content of the combined pill, but no particular group of women have been found to be more or less susceptible to this problem (Fig. 10.7). Furthermore, the BP rise may occur after years of pill use. The mechanism of the hypertensive effect is uncertain and, after stopping the combined pill, high BP may take up to 6 months to return to previous levels [7]. Women who become hypertensive on the combined OC should stop the

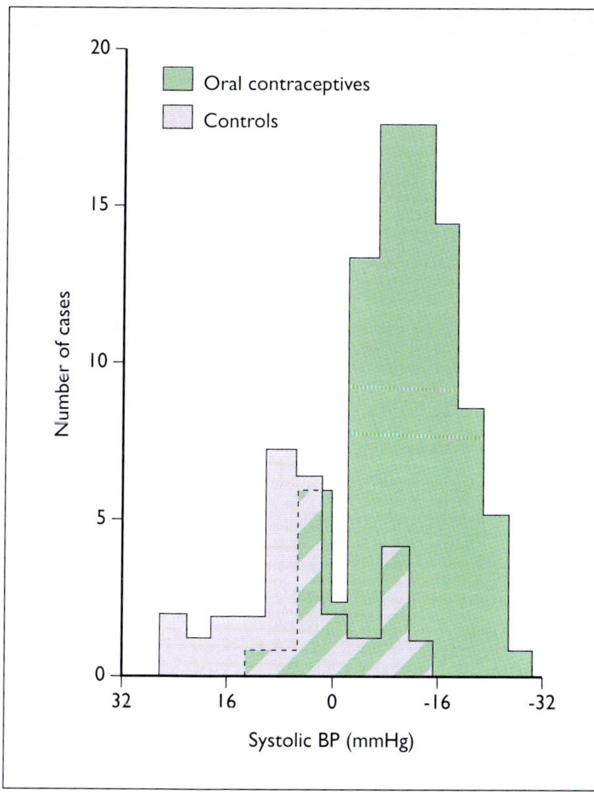

Fig. 10.7 Raised BP in a group of women on an oral contraceptive compared on a group without.

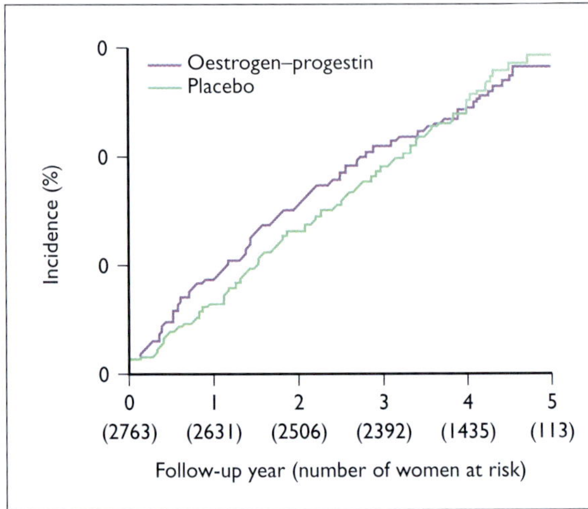

Figure 10.8. Kaplan–Meier estimates of the cumulative incidence of CHD events [8].

OC, particularly if they smoke, suffer from migraine or are over 35 years of age. For women who are reluctant to stop the OC, it is important that their BP is controlled, and the alternative use of a progestogen-only pill (POP) may be helpful. On average the POP does not increase BP, but women rarely have a hypertensive response to it. Close attention to monitoring BP (before starting and 6-monthly thereafter) should be a continuing aspect of managing all forms of oral contraception.

Hormone replacement therapy

Overall, hormone replacement therapy (HRT) in postmenopausal women does not have a significant effect on BP. If there are clear indications for the use of HRT based on troublesome peri- and/or post-menopausal symptoms or osteoporosis risk, the presence of hypertension is not a contraindication. However, a few women may experience a rise in BP consequent to HRT. The anticipated benefits of HRT on overall cardiovascular risk in women that were suggested from observational studies have not been confirmed in the recently published Heart and Estrogen/Progestin Replacement Study (HERS) trial of HRT (Fig. 10.8) in women with established CHD [8].

CHILDREN

BP normally is distributed among children as it is in adults. The tendency of children (and also adults) to remain within their quartile of BP distribution over time is described as tracking. Tracking is tighter for systolic than for diastolic pressure. On average, children of parents with high BP maintain higher levels of BP throughout their development than do those whose parents have normal BP. The factors that influence this relationship are both genetic and those of the shared family environment. Risk factors for hypertension in children are synonymous with those in adults – for instance, infants weaned onto milk feeds with a high salt content have higher BP than those fed on normal breast milk. The associations between obesity, insulin, blood pressure and serum lipids – characterized by insulin resistance in adults – also pertain in children. The familial aggregation of BP and cardiovascular disease (CVD) risk factors offers an important opportunity for primary prevention by identifying the children and adolescents of parents with hypertension.

Measurement technique is particularly important in children and perhaps the most crucial aspect is correct cuff size. The cuff-bladder width should measure approximately 40% of the upper arm circumference. The fifth Korotkoff sound should be used to define diastolic BP for all ages. At the initial evaluation, measurements should be made in both arms and, particularly if high, also in the leg to detect vascular anomalies, including aortic coarctation. The American Task Force on Blood Pressure Control in Children has published means and percentiles of BP relative to age and sex [9]. These detailed tables and graphs take account of both age and height – body size has been identified as the most powerful determinant of BP in children (Fig. 10.9). These data serve to define hypertension in childhood as levels above the 95th percentile (Table 10.5).

High levels of BP among the young make a secondary cause for hypertension more likely. Possible causes of hypertension in infants, children and adolescents are given in Table 10.6. These children may be critically ill at presentation (Table 10.7).

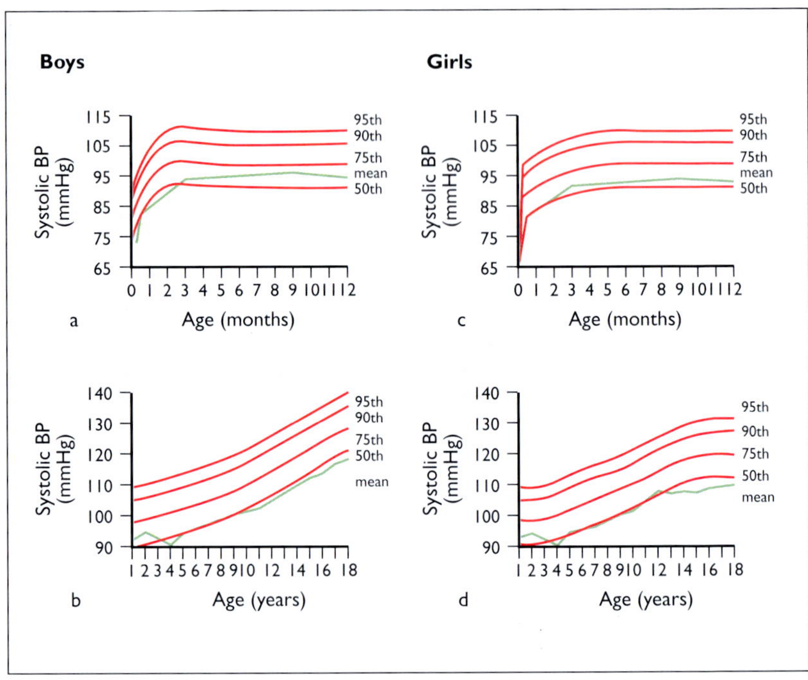

Figure 10.9. Age-specific means and percentiles of systolic BP measurements in children: (a) and (b) boys; (c) and (d) girls [9]. Diastolic BP tracks in similar fashion.

Table 10.5. The 95th percentile of BP at selected ages in girls and boys, by the 50th and 75th height percentiles*

	Percentile for height			
	Girls		Boys	
Age (years)	50th	75th	50th	75th
1	104/58	105/59	102/57	104/58
6	111/73	12/73	114/74	115/75
12	123/80	124/81	123/81	125/82
17	129/84	130/85	136/87	138/88

*Adapted from National High Blood Pressure Education Program [9].

Table 10.6. Secondary causes of hypertension in infants, children and adolescents

Infants	Children and adolescents
■ Coarctation of the aorta	■ Renal parenchymal disease
■ Renal artery thrombosis	■ Renal artery stenosis
■ Renal malformations	■ Coarctation of the aorta
■ Renal parenchymal disease	■ Mineralocorticoid excess
■ Renal artery stenosis	■ Hyperthyroidism
■ Bronchopulmonary dysplasia	■ Phaeochromocytoma
	■ Neurofibromatosis
	■ Neurogenic tumours
	■ Immobilization induced

Table 10.7. Clinical presentation of infants with hypertension

- Congestive heart failure
- Respiratory distress
- Failure to thrive
- Irritability
- Convulsions

For treatment, lifestyle interventions should be strongly recommended. Controlled studies among schoolchildren have shown the potential of lifestyle measures – including diet and exercise – to correct upward trends in BP, weight and cholesterol. This truly amounts to primary prevention – the prevention not simply of events, but of risk factors before they emerge. Drug treatments reflect those used in adults with appropriate dose reductions.

ETHNIC GROUPS

Clinical observations and epidemiological studies indicate important differences in the features of hypertension between various ethnic groups.

Data collated from the *Health Survey for England*, annually performed between 1991 and 1996, and several regional studies in the UK suggest that hypertension is more prevalent amongst African–Caribbeans, although a few earlier surveys, including one of white Europeans, Asians and African–Caribbeans in Birmingham, showed that BPs were equivalent in the three groups. The most striking information comes from the USA, where African–Americans are reported to have the highest prevalence of hypertension in the world [10]. Black patients tend to present with more advanced stages of hypertension and in both countries the debate continues as to whether ethnic differences in hypertension prevalence and control relate to inadequate access to health care among ethnic minorities. Additional observations suggest that correction for other lifestyle differences between blacks and whites – including social class, obesity, dietary factors and physical activity – may account for at least some of the BP differences. Hypertension is not an ancestral problem among blacks in rural Africa, but it is an emerging twenty-first century issue in African towns and cities.

A possible explanation of black susceptibility to hypertension may lie in an impaired ability to excrete sodium. Renal conservation of sodium might have conferred a survival advantage in circumstances in which dietary salt was scarce, but this becomes an adverse attribute if it cannot be downregulated in the setting of salt excess characteristic of westernized diets. This tendency to sodium conservation is associated with low renin levels in black hypertensives and sensitivity to treatment by salt restriction. In addition, black hypertensive patients are probably more responsive to diuretics, calcium antagonists and α-blockers than to β-blockers or ACE inhibitors.

Whether or not black and white ethnic BP differences are predominantly attributable to environmental or genetic factors, black patients suffer more severe consequences of hypertension. In a study that compared untreated black and white hypertensive patients matched for age, sex, BMI, BP and reported duration of hypertension, the black patients had significantly greater LV mass (Fig. 10.10) [11]. Part of the explanation for this greater LVH may be that black patients do not show as great a nocturnal dip in BP as whites. However, further studies have shown that this is not the whole story – there may be a genetic component to the cardiac differences. The pronounced cardiac hypertrophy among black hypertensives might be expected to translate into a higher rate of heart disease mortality, via both coronary events and heart failure. In the USA this does appear to be the case, but in the UK data from the mid 1980s showed lower CHD mortality rates among African–Caribbeans. It is likely that the picture is changing.

It is clear that among all black and Far East Asian (e.g. Chinese) populations, hypertension is more commonly associated with cerebrovascular disease and deteriorating renal function than CHD. In Chinese and Japanese populations, CHD appears to occur less commonly than in European populations. The explanation for these differences is by no means clear, but it appears to relate to the more frequent coexistence in

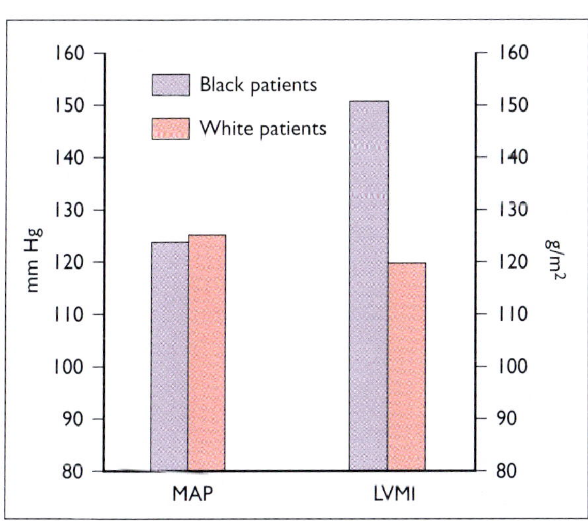

Figure 10.10. Comparison of left ventricular mass index (LVMI) between black and white hypertensive patients with equivalent levels of mean arterial pressure (MAP) and duration of hypertension.

Europeans of additional risk factors for CHD, particularly dyslipidaemia (see Chapter 6). The high stroke rate among blacks is illustrated by comparison of incidence rates of first-ever stroke in USA blacks in Cincinnati with rates in whites in Rochester (Fig. 10.11) [12]; the marked differences at all ages are too great to be plausibly explained by the different locations of the subjects. Hypertension is the strongest of the risk factors for stroke. Also remarkable is the 320% higher rate of hypertension-related end-stage renal disease among African–Americans compared with the rest of the USA population (Fig. 10.12) [13].

In the UK, and in many other parts of the world to which they have migrated, the South Asian population (arising from the Indian subcontinent) is particularly prone to CHD. The classic major risk factors – smoking, BP and serum total cholesterol – do not account for this excess; rather, the other features of insulin resistance and the high

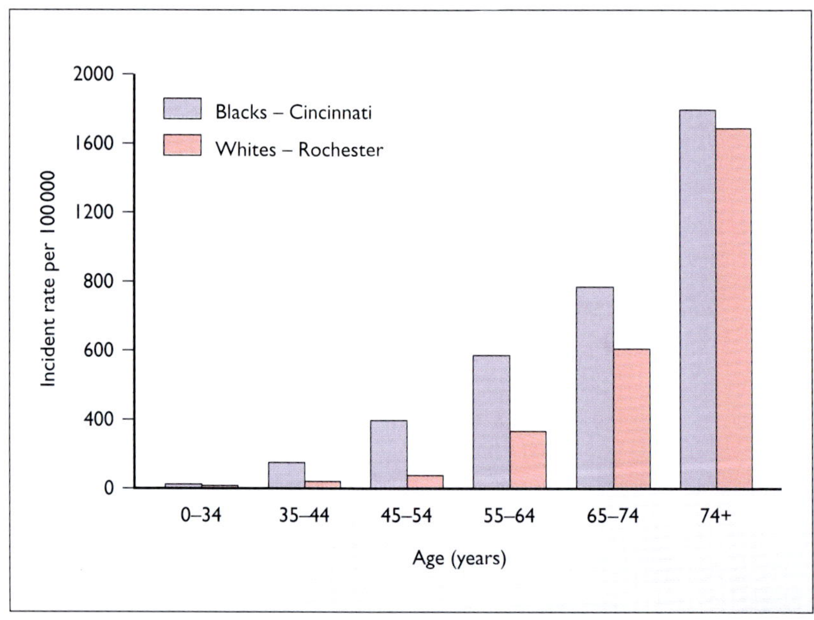

Figure 10.11. Age specific rates for first-ever stroke in black and white populations in the USA [12].

prevalence of diabetes appear to be the reason. Among South Asian diabetics, CHD mortality is particularly high (Fig. 10.13) [14].

In South Asian hypertensives, central obesity, glucose intolerance and dyslipidaemia, particularly low levels of HDL-cholesterol and hypertriglyceridaemia, are common; it is important to consider using antihypertensive drugs that improve this underlying metabolic problem, or at least do not exacerbate it. Hence α-blockers or metabolically neutral agents, may be the preferred therapy in this group, although evidence from randomized controlled trials in South Asians is awaited to confirm or refute this recommendation. Lifestyle advice should concentrate on diet (particularly reduction in saturated cooking fats), smoking cessation, weight loss and increased physical activity – manoeuvres that have been demonstrated to improve insulin resistance [15].

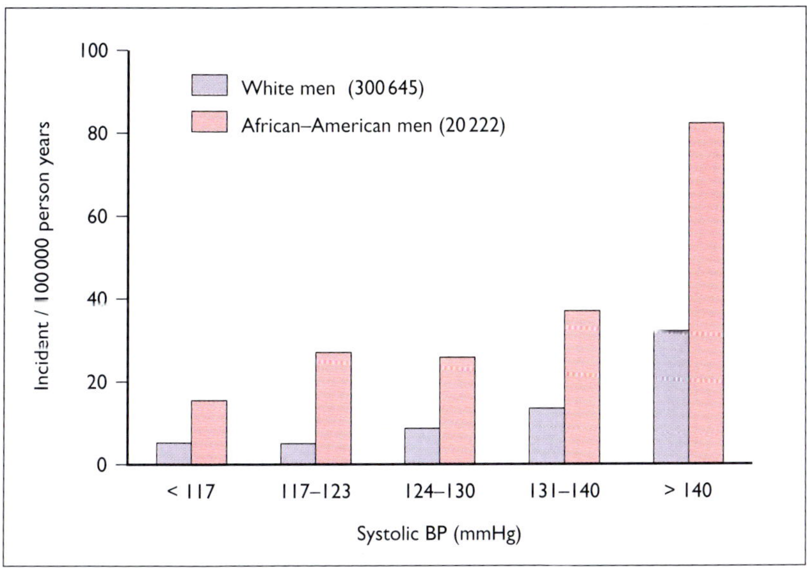

Figure 10.12. Age-adjusted 16-year incidence of all-cause end-stage renal disease by systolic BP amongst black and white men screened for Multiple Risk Factor Intervention Trial [13].

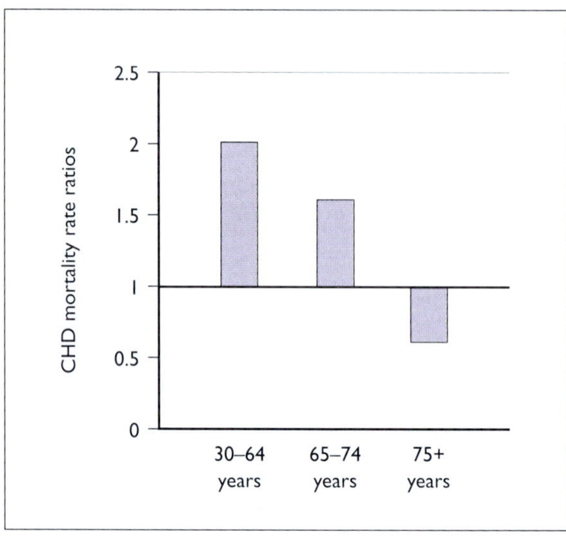

Figure 10.13. Mortality rate ratios for coronary heart disease (South Asian versus European) by age group at baseline among a large cohort of diabetics in West London. The lower mortality in the 75+ years Asians may be a process of selection of residual fitter individuals [14].

Heart Failure

When hypertension is associated with cardiac failure, the resultant morbidity and mortality rates are high. Hypertension (Fig. 10.14) and atherosclerotic CHD are important risk factors for heart failure. Among patients with atrial fibrillation, more than 50% have either current hypertension or a history of hypertension. Hypertension is also a frequent determinant of cardiac arrhythmias – both atrial and ventricular.

Trials of ACE inhibitors have consistently demonstrated improved morbidity and mortality in all grades of heart failure, and delayed progression of cardiac failure in patients with impaired left ventricular function. On the basis of this evidence, ACE inhibitors should be used in the management of the hypertensive patient with either incipient or overt heart failure. However, recent surveys indicate that ACE inhibitors are dramatically underprescribed for patients with clearly defined heart failure, and that when they are used the dosage is usually inadequate [16]. It is important to note that treatment in these trials has almost always been with the combination of ACE inhibitor plus diuretic. The early introduction of diuretics for heart failure is logical because of their combined antihypertensive and natriuretic actions, and their more effective reduction of symptoms. When both agents are used, gradual dose titration is used to avoid precipitous falls in BP.

The efficacy of ACE inhibitors in heart failure emphasizes the advantages of blocking the activated renin–angiotensin–aldosterone axis in heart failure and in hypertension complicated by heart failure. When ACE-inhibitor therapy is indicated, but not tolerated because of side effects (most frequently nonproductive cough), an AII antagonist appears to be a logical alternative. Large trials of AII antagonists in hypertension and heart failure are under way.

Overwhelming evidence now supports the careful use of β-blockers in heart failure. They are most readily applicable to patients with milder symptoms and reasonably maintained ejection fractions. They are not likely to be safe with severely decompensated congestive

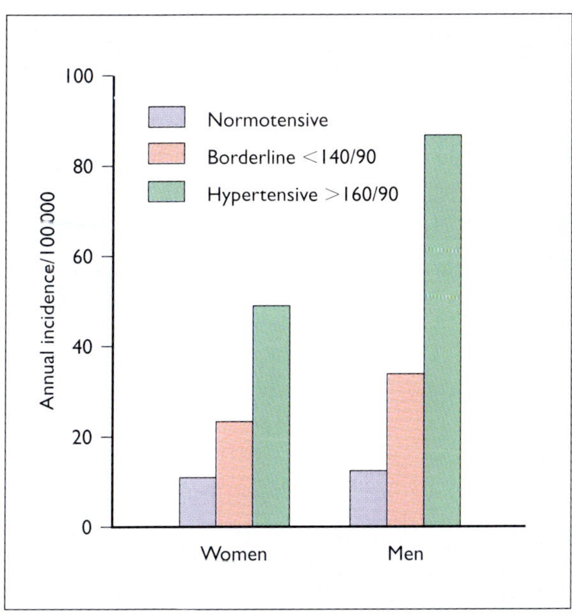

Figure 10.14. Age-adjusted risk of congestive heart failure by hypertension status.

failure – the acute situation needs to be corrected first and left ventricular systolic function ideally assessed by Echo. Treatment needs to be started in low doses and escalated gradually over months to maintenance doses: 'start low and go slow' [17]. The efficacy of β-blockers in heart failure reflects the extreme activation of the sympathetic system – high levels of circulating noradrenaline (norepinephrine) closely track the severity of heart failure. The sympathetic overdrive in this circumstance can be likened to flogging a tired horse to death – function improves with a rest. The β-blockers that have been tested in the largest studies include bisoprolol, metoprolol and carvedilol. Again, combination therapy with ACE inhibitors and diuretics is additive (Fig. 10.15).

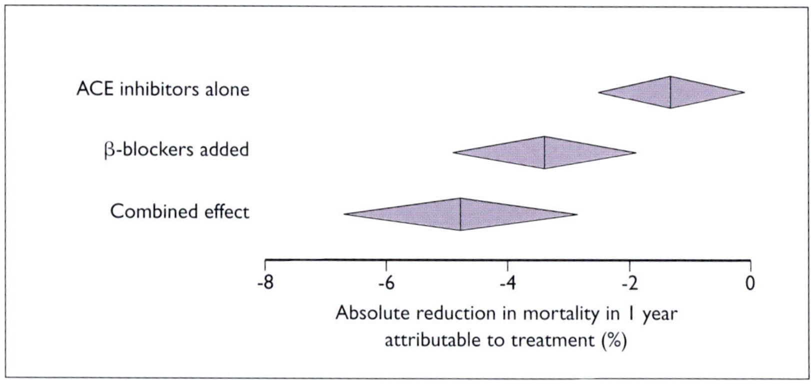

Figure 10.15. Effect on annual rate of mortality (%) of ACE inhibitors alone, with β-blockers added and with both drugs. Risk differences and 95% confidence intervals [17].

Renal impairment

Renal impairment and proteinuria are important indicators of target organ damage and predict diminished survival, as does the presence of LVH. These features should prompt vigorous therapy in the attempt to achieve optimum control at lower target BP.

The combination of hypertension and diabetes frequently causes progressive deterioration in renal function. The key message in both type I and type II diabetes is that BP needs to be treated aggressively with multiple drugs (Table 8.15). Inadequately controlled BP is the strongest determinant of progressive proteinuria and deteriorating renal function in diabetics – the corollary is that the rate of deterioration can be effectively ameliorated with good BP control, however this is achieved. This maxim relates to all forms of renal disease whether or not hypertension was a primary contributor to the pathogenesis of the underlying renal problem. In type I diabetes and in other forms of nephropathy, some evidence indicates that blockade of the renin–angiotensin–aldosterone system offers particular benefit [18] (Fig. 10.16). This may relate to an effective reduction in glomerular hyperfiltration.

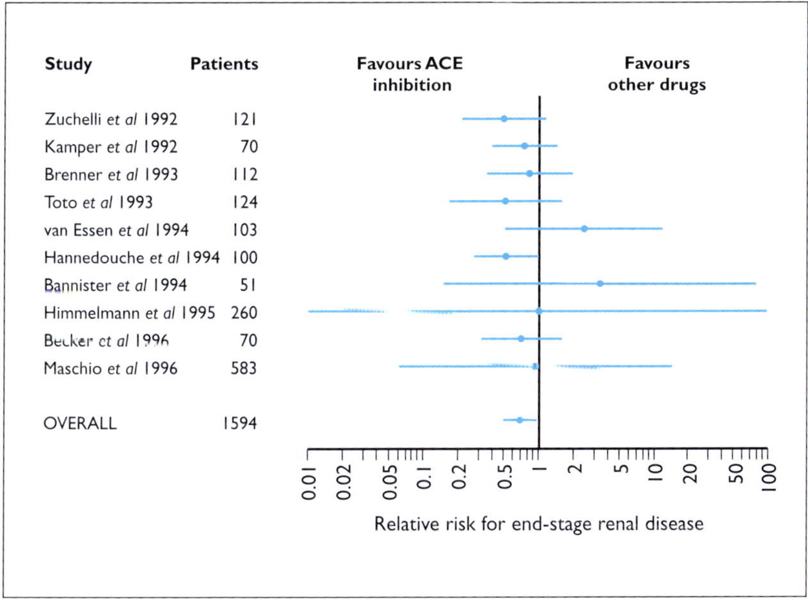

Figure 10.16. Effect of ACE inhibition on risk of end-stage renal disease (ESRD) and death in patients with non-diabetic renal disease [8].

Hypertension may, however, be caused by a primary renal or renovascular pathology; if renal function is deteriorating this may warrant investigation, as different forms of treatment may be necessary. The objective of investigation here is to determine the presence of a correctable cause of hypertension or a treatable primary renal pathology. Several clues to the nature of renal impairment can be found though examination of urine sediment, serological markers of a vasculitic process and noninvasive imaging with ultrasound.

Both ACE inhibitors and AII antagonists should only be used with extreme caution in patients with renal artery stenosis or with severe nephrosclerosis, because there is a risk of precipitating renal failure. With deteriorating levels of glomerular filtration, dosages of antihypertensive drugs that are excreted via the kidneys need adjusting (Table 10.8) [19]. Generally, α-blockers and calcium antagonists can be used without any adjustment in this circumstance.

Resistant hypertension

For patients whose BP is not reasonably controlled on three or more drugs, the causes given in Table 10.9 should be considered.

White-coat hypertension

When high BP, recorded by standard techniques, is subsequently shown by ambulatory measurements to be much lower or even normal, the term white-coat hypertension is used (see Chapter 3). This phenomenon may be apparent to some degree in about one-quarter of patients conventionally labelled as hypertensive [20]. Patients with white-coat hypertension show neither a generalized increase of BP lability, nor an exaggerated pressure response while at work. Although the white-coat effect may be suspected in some patients who appear particularly anxious at the time of examination, and may be accompanied by a tachycardia,

Table 10.8. Antihypertensive drug dosage in chronic renal disease

Drug(%)	Excreted unchanged	Half-life, normal/ ESRD (h)	Dosage % for renal disease GFR (ml/min) >50	10–50x	<10
Diuretic					
Thiazides	>95	6–8/12–20	100	100	Avoid
Frusemide	67	0.5–1.1/2–4	100	100	100
Adrenergic inhibitors					
Peripheral					
Reserpine	<1	46–168/87–323	100	100	Avoid
Central					
Clonidine	45	6–23/39–42	100	100	100
α-blocker					
Doxazosin	<5	9–12/13	100	100	100
β-blocker					
Atenolol	>90	7/15–35	100	50	30–50
Metoprolol	5	3.5/2.5–4.5	100	100	100
Combined α- and β-blockers					
Labetalol	<5	3–9/same	100	100	100
ACE inhibitors					
Captopril	30–40	1.9/21–32	100	75	50
Fosinopril	1	11–12/12–20	100	100	75
Lisinopril	80–90	13/40–50	100	50–75	25–50
Trandolapril	33	10/20	100	75–100	50
A-II receptor blockers					
Losartan	4	6–9/same	100	100	100
CCBs					
Diltiazem	10	2–8/3.5	100	100	100
Verapamil	0	3–7/2–4	100	100	100
Dihydropyridines					
Amlodipine	10	35–50/50	100	100	100
Nifedipine	10	4–6/5–7	100	100	100
Direct vasodilators					
Minoxidil	15–20	3–4/same	100	100	100

Adapted from Bennett *et al* [19].

Table 10.9. Causes of resistant hypertension

- White-coat hypertension
- Noncompliance
- Alcohol excess
- Secondary hypertension
- Obesity
- Nonsteroidal anti-inflammatory drugs
- Sympathomimetics – decongestants, cocaine
- Other drug causes – oral contraceptive pill, corticosteroids, cyclosporin
- Excess salt intake and fluid retention

such features are not always present. The most powerful trigger to the alarm response that underlies this problem is the presence of the doctor (Fig. 10.17). Consequently, many clinics use nurse-recorded BP, although this does not necessarily abolish the alarm response. The magnitude of the 'white-coat' BP increment may be as great as 80/40 mmHg. However, the absence of clinically detectable target organ damage in keeping with sustained hypertension indicates this phenomenon.

The clinical implications of the white-coat response are clearly large and the prevalence of this problem emphasizes the need to take repeated BP recordings at intervals, particularly in those with mild or borderline hypertension [21]. However, its recognition should be balanced by the knowledge that, in the UK, hypertension is adequately controlled by treatment in less than one-quarter of cases. In some patients, the alarm response abates with successive clinic visits and acclimatization to the measurement procedure, but typically, in the genuine white-coat patient, the response remains consistent over repeated visits (Fig. 3.8). Both 24-hour ambulatory measurements of BP or home BP measured by the patient, a relative or a friend often confirm suspicions, as shown in Figure 10.18. However, among those who become hypertensive only

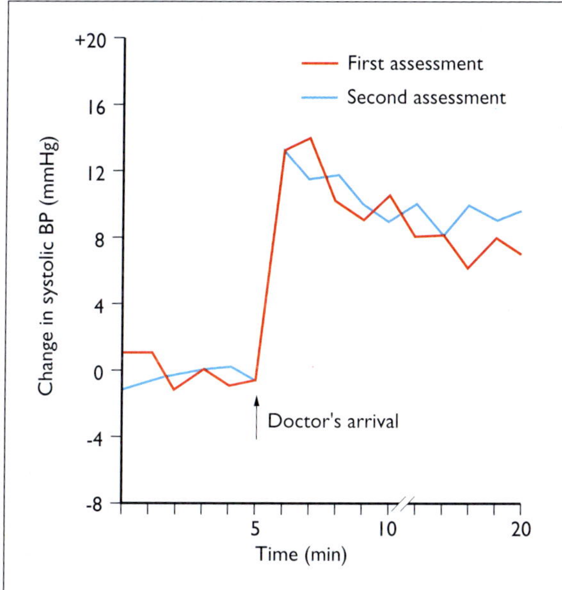

Figure 10.17. Mean BP taken during first and second visits by the same doctor in 35 subjects (See Chapter 3, [4]).

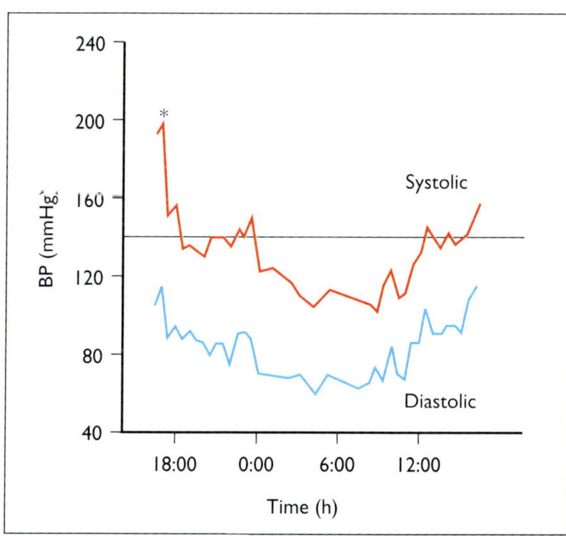

Figure 10.18. Ambulatory BP measurement in a 36-year-old painter and decorator with no target organ damage. (*Measurement made while still in clinic.)

in response to inflation of the measurement cuff, the same problem arises with a standardized 24-hour ambulatory monitoring device. This problem can only be identified by using simultaneous, continuous intra-arterial monitoring and 24-hour ambulatory monitoring!

Casual clinic BP values are, despite their shortcomings, related to cardiovascular mortality and morbidity. It is not yet known how ambulatory measurements relate to these same end-points, although it is evident that 24-hour ambulatory measurements are more closely related to hypertensive cardiovascular structural change than are casual recordings. As stated in Chapter 3, an adjustment factor of 12/7 mmHg needs to be added to the daytime mean BP obtained from ambulatory measurements to give an estimate of the casual clinic equivalent BP.

The problem that confronts the physician is which BP should be used to establish whether or not a patient is hypertensive. We do not know the answer to this question, since all epidemiological studies and intervention trials have been based on casual office measurements of BP. When a significant white-coat component to a patient's BP readings seems likely, it may be reasonable to act in a more conservative way in relation to the introduction of therapy or the escalation of antihypertensive drug treatment. This is, however, an area in which no clear guidelines can be given and one that requires further study. Figure 10.19 offers a pragmatic clinical approach.

All patients with white-coat hypertension should be offered the usual lifestyle advice to prevent high BP and reduce the risk of CVD. If pharmacological treatment is considered for the very anxious patient, it seems logical to use β-blockers, but other drugs, such as verapamil, may be equally effective.

COMPLIANCE

'Compliance' – more recently termed concordance – refers to the extent to which a subject's behaviour in terms of taking medications, dieting or making other lifestyle changes either adheres to or defaults

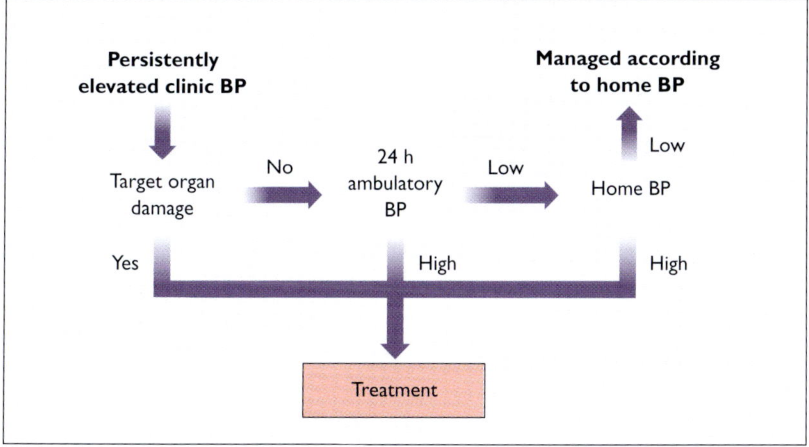

Figure 10.19. Algorithm used to assess true BP if a white-coat effect is suspected.

from medical advice. Poor compliance represents a large therapeutic and economic problem and is one of the most important determinants of efficacy of hypertensive management. It is estimated that 10–15% of patients adhere insufficiently to prescribed drug regimens. In the special Veterans Administration hypertension clinics, a 38% drop-out rate had occurred after 6 years' follow-up. In relation to the rule of halves in hypertension detection and control, this problem must account for a high proportion of the 50% of all hypertensives who are treated and yet uncontrolled.

The many contributory aspects to compliance problems include forgetfulness, poor understanding of complex regimens, inadequate explanation provided by the doctor, prohibitive costs of medications or prescription charges, fear of adverse side effects and the expectation that hypertension will be cured after a short course of treatment. Many of these reflect poor communication between the doctor and the patient but, above all, it is difficult to persuade asymptomatic patients to take life long medication without absolute assurance of benefit. This is particularly emphasized by the observation that patients are more likely to feel worse than better after diagnosis of hypertension and initiation of treatment.

Data from the Medical Research Council indicate that side effects are a major problem with some first-line therapies – approximately 20% of the subjects in the β-blocker and diuretic groups were withdrawn from treatment because of side effects, whereas only about 5% were withdrawn from the placebo group.

Uncertainties about compliance complicate the physician's interpretation of progress since the patient's clinical response may result from any one of four interactions between compliance and efficacy (Table 10.10). Misclassification causes problems, such as when noncompliance is unsuspected, the response low/poor is incorrectly assumed to be the response high/poor and the physician may prescribe additional medication. If the newly increased therapy is taken as prescribed, perhaps during hospitalization, severe hypotension may result.

Various techniques have been used to try to measure compliance. The most direct involves measurement of drug or metabolites in urine, but such assays are expensive and not readily available. Individual

Table 10.10. Interactions between compliance and efficacy of management of hypertension

- **High/good** (high compliance with good BP control achieved) – describing the ideal situation of correct diagnosis, full patient adherence and complete pharmacological response
- **High/poor** (high compliance, without BP control) – suggesting an inappropriate treatment, insufficent dosage or pharmacological resistance
- **Low/good** (low compliance, with BP control achieved) – indicative of incorrect initial diagnosis in a subject not needing antihypertensive treatment at all
- **Low/poor** (low compliance, without BP control) – corresponding to the typical noncompliant patient

methods include patient self-monitoring (aided by blister packaging of tablets), pill counts at clinic visits and frequency of prescription refills. These are all unreliable as many factors can influence the assessments.

The automatic medication monitor represents a recent sophisticated advance, although to date such devices have only been used in trial circumstances. This device lies in the container lid and records the frequency and precise time of opening of the medication vial. The presumption is that once the lid is opened and the medication dispensed, the tablet is taken.

In practice, the presence or absence of drug-associated symptoms, metabolic changes or clinical signs (e.g. bradycardia in patients on β-blockers) may be a useful guide.

Doctors resort to many ploys to enhance compliance when a problem is suspected. These frequently involve veiled threats by generating fear of the consequences of uncontrolled hypertension. However, fear does not often appear to be an effective inducement to comply.

Studies have reported that the approaches shown in Table 10.11 increase compliance.

Table 10.11. Measures that increase compliance with antihypertensive therapy

- Increasing the quality of instructions
- Ensuring that the patient understands the reasons for treatment
- Dealing with difficult aspects of multicomponent therapy one at a time
- Simplifying drug regimens to avoid midday dosing, preferably achieving once-daily dosing
- Putting treatment regimens and objectives in writing
- Being friendly, courteous and compassionate
- Facilitating patients' opportunities for questions and discussion, and enhancing participation in their own care
- Responding sensitively to complaints

EXCESS ALCOHOL INTAKE

Early observations regarding alcohol and BP (Fig. 4.10) [22] have been confirmed by many epidemiological studies, which have shown that higher levels of alcohol intake are associated with higher rates of hypertension (Fig. 10.20). On average, those individuals who consume more than 21 units of alcohol per week have higher levels of BP, and those who drink six or more drinks per day are twice as likely to develop hypertension. Very high alcohol consumption can produce a marked elevation of BP; clinical case reports describe a phaeochromocytoma-like syndrome (pseudophaeochromocytoma). The mechanisms by which alcohol induces higher levels of BP have not been identified, but it is likely that obesity and sympathetic overactivity almost certainly contribute. In addition to adverse effects on body weight, excess alcohol intake may induce adverse

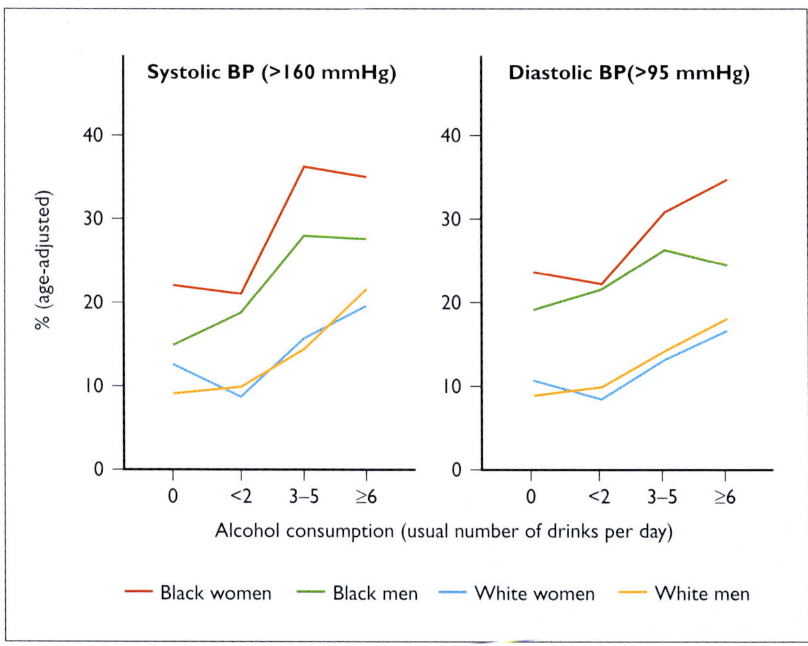

Figure 10.20. Increase in hypertension prevalence with alcohol intake: 1977 study.

effects on lipid profiles, particularly by producing elevated triglyceride levels, although HDL cholesterol is increased.

Reduced alcohol consumption often results in lower BP levels, and in some patients may be the only intervention required. Hence, it is important to establish whether alcohol is playing an important role in hypertension. Abnormal liver enzymes, γGTP and a raised mean MCV may provide clues to excess alcohol intake (which is often denied).

Largely because of variations in alcohol consumption, mean BP levels of the general population vary throughout the week, being highest over the weekend and on Monday. The practical implication of this observation is to avoid measuring critical BP levels only on a Monday morning in those suspected of weekend binge drinking. Given the 'cardioprotective' effects of alcohol against ischaemic heart disease (Fig. 10.21), patients should not necessarily be told to stop alcohol consumption (unless they are alcoholics), but rather to moderate intake [23,24]. Realistic, practical advice to switch to low-alcohol beers and to 'water down' wine with soda water should be supplied, particularly for those whose social life revolves around the pub. Alcohol-induced hypertension is notably resistant to drug treatment – no specific drug group has been demonstrated to be particularly effective in these patients, although β-blockers may be a logical choice if sympathetic hyperactivity is involved as a pathogenic mechanism.

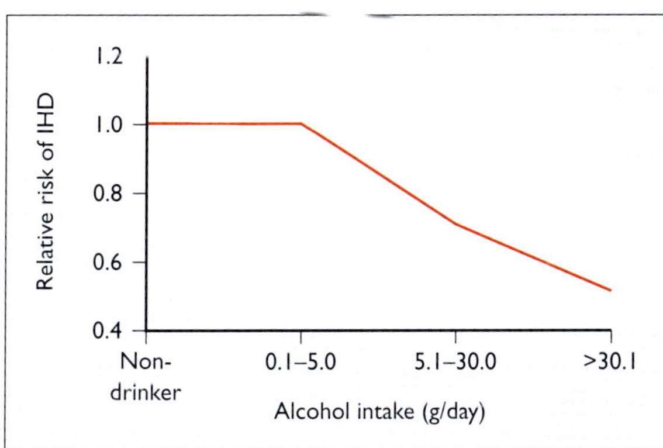

Figure 10.21. Relative risks of ischaemic heart disease (IHD) with alcohol consumption (health professionals study; 44 059 men followed over 2 years; 1 unit of alcohol = 8 g) [22].

SECONDARY CAUSES OF HYPERTENSION

General issues

Secondary causes of hypertension probably account for less than 5% of all cases of hypertension (Fig. 10.22). Clues that a secondary cause for hypertension may be present are given in Table 10.12. Diagnosis of these secondary causes relies on the recognition of specific clinical features (Table 10.12) and signs, and aspects of the history that should prompt further investigations (Table 10.13). In addition, a careful drug history should reveal the possible influence of a variety of drugs – the combined contraceptive pill, nonsteroidal anti-inflammatories, liquorice, corticosteroids and recreational drugs such as cocaine and amphetamines.

The interpretation of a positive or negative family history of hypertension is difficult. On the one hand the high prevalence of essential hypertension means that many individuals with an underlying secondary cause concurrently have a positive family history and, on the other hand, some of the secondary causes of hypertension have a familial linkage. A few simple, inexpensive investigations can be regarded as screening tests

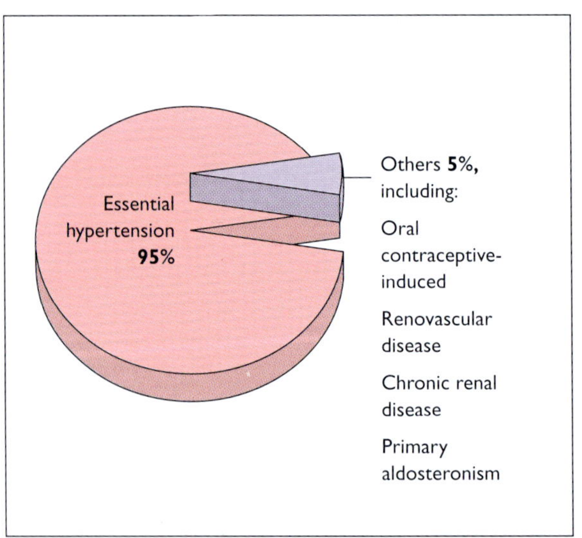

Figure 10.22. Frequency of secondary causes of hypertension.

(e.g. plasma sodium and potassium). Beyond this, the use of definitive investigations must be driven by clinical suspicion.

A proposed simple algorithm for the investigation of hypertension in relation to possible secondary causes in given in Figure 10.23.

Table 10.12. Clues to secondary causes of hypertension

Symptom	Condition
Thirst, polyuria, nocturia	Chronic renal disease, diabetes, hyperparathyroidism
Loin pain, colic	Analgesic nephropathy, pyelonephritis, polycystic disease, renal artery stenosis
Haematuria, oedema	Glomerulonephritis
Muscle weakness	Conn's syndrome
Postural hypotension	Phaeochromocytoma, Conn's syndrome
Palpitations, sweating, paroxysmal headache	Phaeochromocytoma

Table 10.13. Indications for further investigation

- Clinical features of an underlying cause (see Table 10.12)
- Onset before age 30 years
- Rapid progression
- Proteinuria, haematuria, glycosuria
- Severe hypertension; difficult to control
- Vascular disease – peripheral, carotid, coronary
- Heart failure

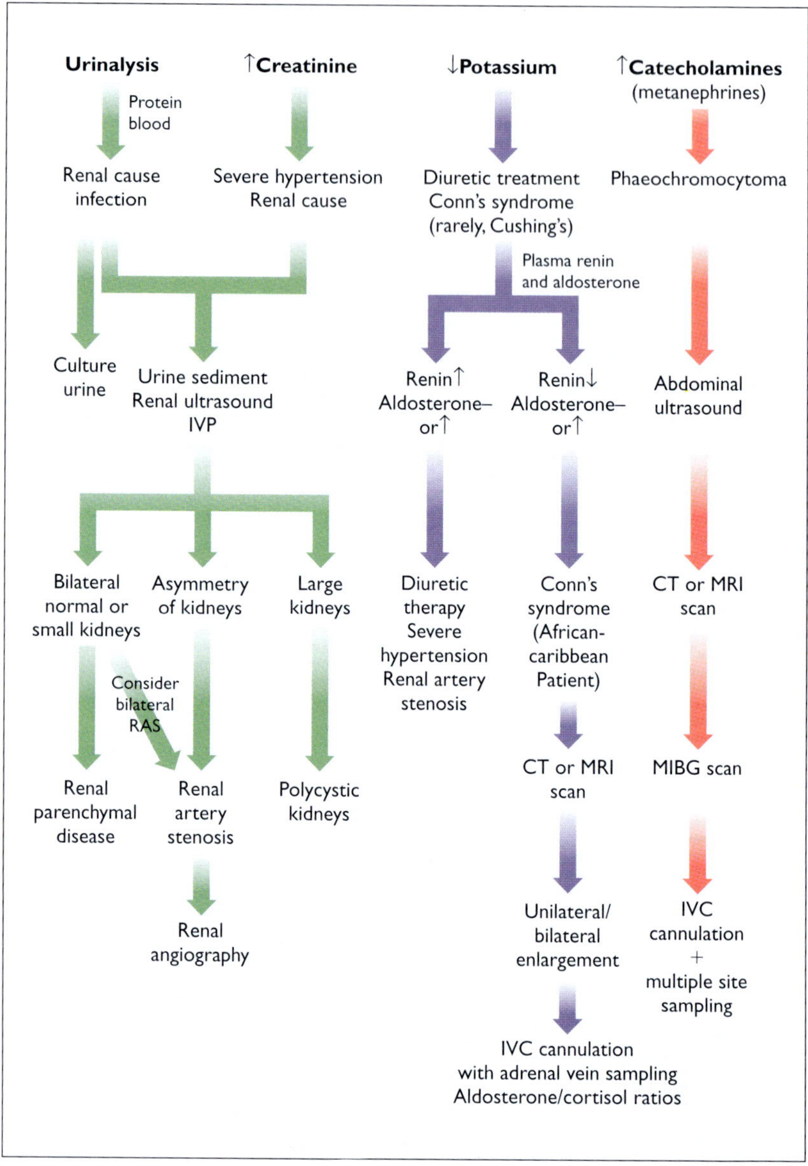

Figure 10.23. Algorithm for investigation of secondary causes of hypertension. IVC, inferior vena cava; IVP, intravenous pyelogram; MIBG, mono-iodo-benzyl guanidine; RAS, renal artery stenosis.

Phaeochromocytoma

Phaeochromocytoma is a rare cause of hypertension. In the classic patient, hypertension is paroxysmal and associated with typical symptoms of headache, palpitations and a sensation of anxiety caused by catecholamine excess. Sustained hypertension in the absence of such symptoms may rarely be associated with an underlying adrenal tumour. Although these tumours, which secrete noradrenalin and adrenalin (norepinephrine and epinephrine), may occasionally be bilateral, very occasionally malignant and found outside the adrenal gland, they are usually localized within the adrenal gland, unilateral and benign. Phaeochromocytoma may be associated with von Recklinghausen's disease, which is a familial condition associated with multiple neurofibromatosis and café-au-lait skin lesions. The patient with phaeochromocytoma is at grave risk of a vascular catastrophe and may present with the consequences of vasospastic ischaemia, such as angina.

The preferred screening investigations include measurements of 24-hour urine catecholamines or the metabolites, normetanephrine and metanephrine. Plasma catecholamine measurements are also highly sensitive, but the traditional measurement of urinary VMA is unreliable and lacks sensitivity and specificity. Pharmacological provocation tests should be abandoned as they are nonspecific and hazardous. The tumours may be localized by ultrasound techniques, computed tomography (CT) or magnetic resonance imaging (MRI). Localization by radionuclide scans or angiography is sometimes indicated, particularly for extra-adrenal tumours.

The treatment for phaeochromocytoma is excision of the tumour, which should be carried out in a specialized centre with experience of such cases, as the anaesthetic and operative procedures are hazardous. Prior to surgery, good BP control is best achieved using a nonselective α-blocker in combination with a β-blocker (e.g. phenoxybenzamine and atenolol). β-blockers may be necessary to control palpitations, but should not be introduced prior to α-blockers lest hypertensive surges are exacerbated. Acute elevations in BP during surgery may need parenteral therapy with phentolamine or labetalol.

Conn's syndrome

Primary hyperaldosteronism, or Conn's syndrome, is increasingly recognized as a cause of hypertension. It results from excessive quantities of aldosterone being produced by one or both adrenal cortices. The classic distinction of unilateral adenoma from bilateral adrenal hyperplasia is almost certainly an oversimplification and represents two extremes of a continuum of pathology. The diagnosis may be suspected by the finding of hypokalaemia on routine screening of a hypertensive patient. Primary hyperaldosteronism is invariably associated with a high–normal serum sodium (>140 mmol/l). Hypokalaemia is often exposed or exacerbated by the introduction of diuretic therapy, which induces a more dramatic fall in the serum potassium than would otherwise be considered normal. Occasionally, this may be sufficiently severe to produce symptoms of profound fatigue. In the untreated patient, supportive evidence for a diagnosis of hyperaldosteronism may be suggested by the finding of a suppressed plasma renin and a high or high–normal circulating aldosterone, but these are, however, poorly predictive. However, an aldosterone: renin ratio in excess of 750 improves the predictive value. Importantly, drug treatment of hypertension may markedly influence the levels of these hormones, with suppression of renin by β-blockers and elevation of renin by diuretics, ACE inhibitors and AII antagonists. When Conn's syndrome is

Table 10.14. Example of biochemical values in Conn's syndrome

Test	Typical value
Na↑	145mmol/l
K↓	3.0 mmol/l
Renin↓	0.2 pmol/ml/hr
Aldosterone↑	790 pmol/l

suspected, referral to a specialist centre is advised, where investigation involves attempted localization of a single benign adenoma with ultrasound, CT or MRI. Radionuclide studies using radiolabelled cholesterol, preferably carried out with prior dexamethasone suppression, may indicate whether there is unilateral or bilateral hyperactivity of the adrenal glands.

The definitive treatment of unilateral disease is adrenalectomy. Attempts at adrenal ablation using sclerosing techniques have been successful in a number of cases. It is advisable, in most cases in which surgery is contemplated, to undertake further studies with inferior vena caval catheterization and bilateral adrenal vein sampling for aldosterone and cortisol ratios, to establish beyond doubt whether the excess aldosterone secretion is unilateral or bilateral.

The treatment for bilateral disease is with drugs that competitively antagonize or inhibit the action of aldosterone on the distal tubule, such as spironolactone and amiloride, respectively. Control of BP may require the addition of a calcium antagonist, which complements the actions of anti-aldosterone therapy.

Renal artery stenosis

Renal artery stenosis probably accounts for less than 2% of the total hypertensive population. However, in patients with accelerated hypertension the prevalence is much higher – up to 43% in whites and 7% in blacks.

Two distinct pathological types of stenosis occur. The first is fibromuscular hyperplasia, which is an accumulation or a disorganization of fibrous material arising from the intima or media of the arterial wall that encroaches on the lumen. Typically, this occurs as alternating bands of narrowing and dilatation, giving rise to a 'string of beads' appearance on angiography (Fig. 10.24) or, alternatively, as localized regions of concentric narrowing (Fig. 10.25). The aetiology of this condition is uncertain. It is frequently bilateral and may be associated with a similar process in the carotid arteries and other visceral arteries. The condition arises in young patients, most commonly in younger, white women.

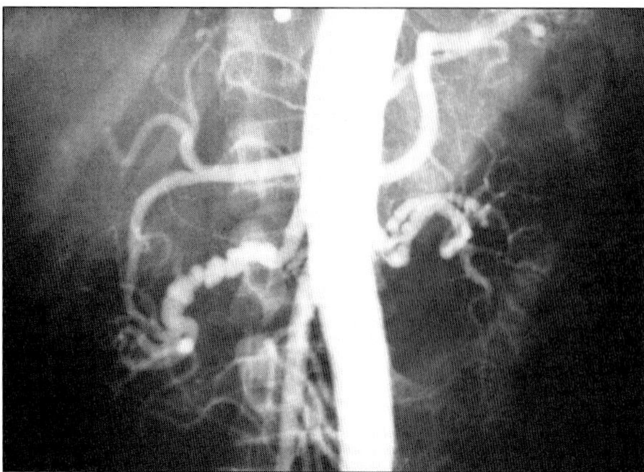

Figure 10.24. Fibromuscular renal artery stenosis with a 'string of beads' appearance.

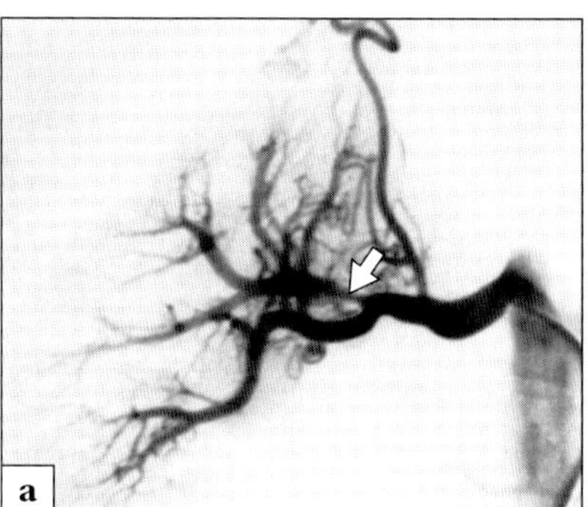

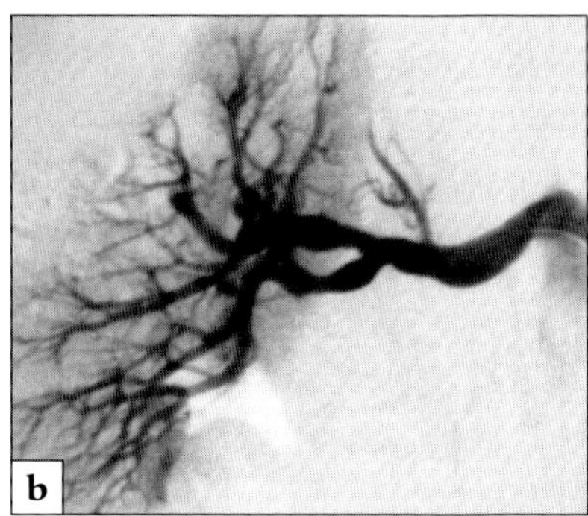

Figure 10.25. Fibromuscular renal artery stenosis: focal concentric (arrow) narrowing before (a) and after (b) balloon angioplasty.

The second type is atheromatous renal artery disease, which causes hypertension when atheromatous deposits narrow the artery lumen. The lesions frequently involve the ostia of the renal arteries (Fig. 10.26), with atheromatous plaques that extend from the aortic wall. Otherwise they occur within the proximal part of the artery and are bilateral in 25% of cases. The patient is most typically a middle-aged male smoker with evidence of concurrent atheromatous disease at other sites. It is evident that atheromatous renovascular disease shares the same risk factors as

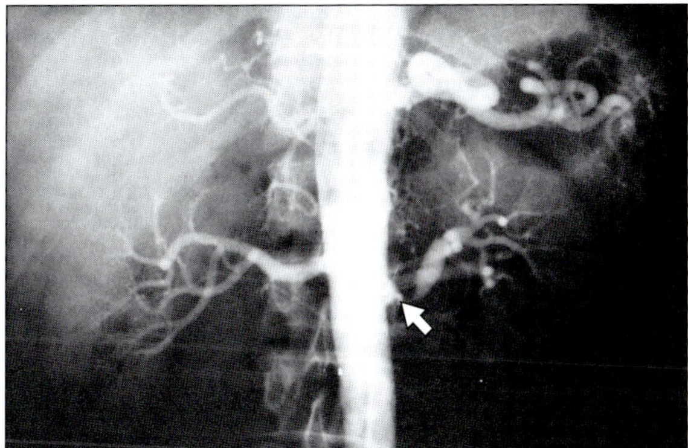

Figure 10.26. Atheromatous renal artery stenosis (arrow).

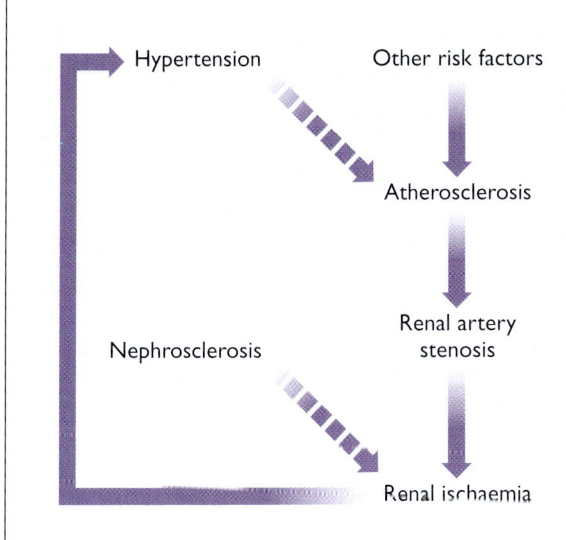

Figure 10.27. Interrelationship between hypertension and renal disease.

atheroma elsewhere; it is often difficult to be sure which came first – the hypertension or the renal artery stenosis (Fig. 10.27). However, there may be a well-documented deterioration in BP control accompanied (particularly in bilateral disease) by a rising creatinine level. This renal impairment may be rapidly accelerated by the use of ACE inhibitors.

Hypertension driven by renal artery stenosis is in part renin dependent, so a dramatic fall in BP accompanied by a rise in creatinine after treatment with an ACE inhibitor or AII antagonist should prompt diagnosis. Either condition may be accompanied by a renal artery bruit, but this is not a reliable sign. Estimation of plasma renin activity is a useful screening test, but only has moderate sensitivity and specificity. The current definitive investigation is direct catheter angiography, but MRI with blood flow evaluations promises to be a sensitive noninvasive technique.

Treatment objectives differ in the two conditions. In fibromuscular hyperplasia the goal is cure of the hypertension, which can be achieved in about 60% of cases with some BP improvement in most of the rest. The lesions are best corrected by balloon angioplasty and have a low recurrence rate. In atheromatous disease, the treatment objective is principally preservation of renal function and secondary improvement of BP control. Atheromatous lesions have a high recurrence rate after angioplasty. The outcome may be improved by the use of satins, aspirin, intraluminal stenting, or reconstructive surgery may be required. With the exception of ACE inhibitors and AII antagonists, which are contraindicated in this condition, the choice of antihypertensive agent need not be directly influenced by the underlying pathology. The severity and refractory nature of the BP often requires three drugs used in combination.

Essential hypertension

Having excluded as far as possible the other causes of resistant hypertension described in this chapter, the remaining diagnosis of exclusion is severe essential hypertension. This condition demands effective management because of the associated high mortality rates.

Attempts to lower BP should begin immediately, but the rate of BP fall should not be too rapid. The use of non-pharmacological measures should always be encouraged since, even though these may not in themselves have a major impact on BP, they are likely to result in fewer and/or lower doses of drugs being necessary. After initiating therapy with one or two drugs at low doses, each drug should be titrated to produce optimal efficacy with minimal side effects before adding in the next drug.

Patients with severe hypertension frequently require at least three drugs. The standard regimen of 'triple therapy' – diuretic plus β-blocker plus vasodilator – is often effective in terms of BP lowering. However, the availability of newer agents has given rise to the combination of ACE inhibitor plus calcium antagonist plus α-blocker, which is extremely effective and appears to offer some advantages over triple therapy in terms of metabolic profile and effects on other surrogate end-points. Diuretics (sometimes in the form of spironolactone) make a suitable fourth-line agent if this newer three-drug combination remains ineffective.

When fourth- and fifth-line agents are required, the use of minoxidil may become necessary. At low doses (e.g. 5 mg twice a day), this drug is reasonably well tolerated, although hirsutism, particularly for women, and oedema are common side effects.

It is important to ensure that the patient understands the regimen; hence, for simplicity, different dosing frequencies should be avoided by using a once-daily regimen for all drugs, if possible. Failure to do so frequently results in inadvertent noncompliance. As more drugs, with more side effects, fail to control BP, the patients may also be more prone to a white-coat effect superimposed on their genuine condition and failing compliance. Only careful BP monitoring (including 24-hour measurements), reassurance and supervised drug management can help to disentangle the possible causes of severe resistant hypertension in such cases.

CHAPTER SUMMARY

- The special situations discussed in this chapter are relatively rare in primary care and, therefore, a shared-care protocol has an important role to play.
- Good communication with the secondary-care sector is essential when managing these patients.
- In the elderly, BP thresholds for initiating treatment remain the same as in younger patients; target BP also remains the same.
- Pregnancy planning is essential for hypertensive mothers – with adequate care and supervision there is a good chance of a successful outcome. Both the PHCT and the obstetric team need to be closely involved at an early stage.
- Close attention to monitoring BP should be a continuing aspect of managing all forms of contraception.
- Overall, HRT does not have a significant effect on BP, but there are important exceptions to this generalization.
- Measurement technique is particularly important in children; hypertension in this group is more likely to arise from a secondary cause.
- There are important differences in the features of hypertension between various ethnic groups.
- If hypertension is associated with cardiac failure, the resultant morbidity and mortality rates are high.
- Renal impairment and proteinuria are important indicators of target organ damage and predict diminished survival.
- In patients whose BP is not reasonably controlled on three or more drugs, consider why.
- A white-coat response may contribute to BP readings in both normotensive and hypertensive individuals.

- Poor compliance represents a large therapeutic and economic problem.
- High levels of alcohol intake are associated with hypertension which is often labile.
- Secondary causes of hypertension account for less than 5% of all cases of hypertension.
- When secondary causes are suspected, referral is recommended.
- Severe essential hypertension demands effective management.
- Patients with severe hypertension frequently require three or more drugs.
- The newer drugs may offer some advantages in terms of metabolic profile and surrogate end points. Trials to evaluate benefits on morbidity and mortality are in progress.

References

1. Westerhof N, O'Rourke MF. Haemodynamic basis for the development of left ventricular failure in systolic hypertension and for its logical therapy. *J Hypertens* 1995; **13**: 943–52.
2. Mitchell GF, Moye LA, Braunwald E *et al.* Sphygmomanometrically determined pulse pressure is a powerful independent predictor of recurrent events after myocardial infarction in patients with impaired left ventricular function. SAVE investigators. *Circulation*. 1997; **96**: 4254–60.
3. World Health Report 1977. http://www.who.org/whr/1997/factse.htm.
4. Cappuccio FP, Markandu ND, Carney C, Sagnella GA, MacGregor GA. Double-blind randomised trial of modest salt restriction in older people. *Lancet* 1997; **350**: 850–54.
5. National High Blood Pressure Education Program. Working group report on high blood pressure in pregnancy. *Am J Obstet Gynecol* 1990; **163**: 1689–712.
6. Redman CWG, Beilin LJ, Bonnar J, Ounsted MK. Fetal outcome in trial of anti-hypertensive treatment in pregnancy. *Lancet* 1976; **ii**: 753–6.
7. Weir RJ, Briggs E, Mack A, Naismith L, Taylor L, Wilson E. Blood pressure in women taking oral contraceptives. *Br Med J* 1974; **i**: 533–5.
8. Hulley S, Grady D, Bush T, *et al.* Randomized trial of estrogen plus progestin for secondary prevention of coronary heart disease in postmenopausal women. *JAMA* 1998; **280**: 605–13.
9. National High Blood Pressure Education Program. Working group on hypertension control in children and adolescents. *Pediatrics* 1996; **98**: 649–58.
10. Burt VL, Whelton P, Roccella EJ, *et al.* Prevalence of hypertension in the US adult population: results from the third National Health and Nutrition Examination Survey, 1988–1991. *Hypertension* 1995; **25**: 305–13.
11. Mayet J, Shahi M, Foale RA, Poulter NR, Sever PS, Thom SMcG. Racial differences in cardiac structure and function in essential hypertension. *Br Med J* 1994; **308**: 1011–4.
12. Broderick J, Brott T, Kothari R, *et al.* The Greater Cincinnati/Northern Kentucky Stroke Study: preliminary first-ever and total incidence rates of stroke among blacks. *Stroke* 1998; **29**: 415–21.
13. Klag MJ. End-stage renal disease in African–American and white men. 16-year MRFIT findings. *JAMA*. 1997; **277**: 1293–8.

14. Mather HM, Chaturvedi N, Fuller JH. Mortality and morbidity from diabetes in South Asians and Europeans: 11-year follow-up of the Southall diabetes survey, London, UK. *Diabet Med* 1998; **15**: 53–9.
15. Kooner JS. Coronary heart disease in UK Indian Asians: the potential for reducing mortality. *Heart* 1997; **78**: 5302.
16. Hood S, Taylor S, Hemingway H. Older patients and advances in cardiology. *Lancet* 1997; **350**: 1779–80.
17. Cleland JGF, McGowan J, Clark A. The evidence for β-blockers in heart failure. *Br Med J* 1999; **318**: 824–5.
18. Giatras I, Lau J, Levey AS. Effect of angiotensin-converting enzyme inhibitors on the progression of non-diabetic renal disease: a meta-analysis of randomized trials. *Ann Intern Med* 1997; **127**: 337–45.
19. Bennet WM, Aronoff GR, Golpher TA, *et al. Drug Prescribing in Renal Failure. Dose Guidelines for Adults*. Philadelphia: American College of Physicians, 1994.
20. Pickering TG, James GD, Boddie C, Harshfield GA, Blank S, Laragh JH. How common is white coat hypertension? *JAMA* 1988; **259**: 225–8.
21. O'Brien E, O'Malley K. Overdiagnosing hypertension. *Br Med J* 1988; **297**: 1211–2.
22. Lian C. L'alcoolisme, cause d'hypertension arterielle. *Bull Acad Natl Med* 1915; **74**: 525–8.
23. Rimm EB, Giovannucci EL, Willett WC, *et al.* Prospective study of alcohol consumption and risk of coronary disease in men. *Lancet* 1991; **338**: 464–8.
24. Rimm EB, Klatsky A, Grobbee D, Stampfer MJ, *et al.* Review of moderate alcohol consumption and reduced risk of coronary heart disease: is the effect due to beer, wine, or spirits? *Br Med J* 1996; **312**: 731–6.

chapter 11

Case histories

CASE 1

A 76-year-old man has recovered from a recent small stroke (after which he gave up smoking). He is at least 15 kg overweight, and 4 years previously he suffered a transient ischaemic attack (TIA) characterized by transient dysphasia. One week after the small recent stroke his BP was 190/130 mmHg with grade II retinopathy, and urine dipstix showed 2+ proteinuria plus. Treatment is initiated gradually. The following week, BP is 137/85 mmHg, there is 2+ protein and 2+ blood in the urine. The creatinine has risen from 120 to 197 mmol/l.

- What are your treatment objectives here?
- At what stage would you initiate antihypertensive therapy after a stroke, and what are your concerns?
- What other information would you like to assist your management?
- Why do you think the serum creatinine has risen?
- What other possible issues need to be considered?
- What further steps will you take?

Discussion

Treatment objectives

The treatment objectives are to prevent further strokes and to correct risk factors for CVD overall. CHD is still the most likely cause of death in patients who have suffered strokes. This man has already achieved major benefit by stopping smoking.

Treating poststroke hypertension

The time at which to initiate antihypertensive treatment after stroke is a difficult issue because the pressure–flow relationship in the severe hypertensive (and post-stroke) cerebral circulation is shifted upwards. Thus the pressure range across which the cerebral circulation is able to 'autoregulate' constant flow is higher. Consequently, the magnitude of BP reduction achieved in this man may prove disastrous in terms of extending the stroke, particularly if the pressure is dropped acutely. This difficult and common clinical problem is currently the focus of an intervention trial. The current consensus is to wait for 10 days after an event before initiating antihypertensive treatment gradually. With extremely severe BP levels (>220/130 mmHg) the risk of haemorrhage warrants cautious and gradual reduction of BP at an earlier stage. It may be that certain antihypertensive agents (ACE inhibitors) have an advantage in that they maintain cerebral autoregulation in this circumstance.

The patient's marked fall in BP in response to gradual treatment may have a number of explanations. Firstly, acute hypertension associated with stroke may tend to settle spontaneously. However, the 53/45 mmHg reduction associated with a rise in creatinine suggests that the man may have renovascular disease and that an ACE inhibitor has been used. If so, the ACE inhibitor should be discontinued – instead a β-blocker and calcium antagonist combination may prove effective and safer from a renal point of view. Alternatively, the BP fall (and the creatinine rise) may relate to myocardial infarction-induced hypotension occurring in this acutely stressful interval. Vascular disease that presents in one location in a multirisk patient is invariably associated with disease at other critical sites.

Further information required

Further information is required about this patient's cardiac function both in terms of stroke causation and cardiovascular risk. For stroke causation the following need to be ascertained:

- Is he in atrial fibrillation? Could the fall in BP have been precipitated by arrhythmia?
- Is there evidence of previous myocardial infarction? Is there a probability of mural thrombus? Would an Echo be useful (often it would)?
- Are there any cardiac murmurs or signs of endocarditis? The presence of haematuria and proteinuria in association with a stroke raises this possibility. Equally, the possibility of another form of vasculitis should be considered (determining the erythrocyte sedimentary rate should be part of a preliminary stroke screen). Other more common but possibly coincidental urological causes of haematuria and proteinuria should also be considered (prostatic disease, bladder infection, bladder tumour).
- Is there any cardiac indication of septal defect and paradoxical embolism? This anomaly, which is surprisingly common, needs consideration particularly in the younger individual with no obvious vascular risk factors.

In terms of future cardiovascular risk, the following information is required:
- Is there evidence of longstanding hypertension – LVH on the ECG or Echo? The grade II retinopathy indicates probable longstanding hypertension.
- Are there additional risk factors? What is the cholesterol profile? Is he diabetic?

Further information about the nature of the stroke is useful. Generally, in Europe and the USA, about 80% of strokes are thrombotic or thromboembolic, with most of the remainder being intracerebral haemorrhage. However, the proportion of haemorrhagic strokes is higher with higher levels of BP and with younger age. The past history of TIA in this patient and the relatively rapid recovery indicate that this recent stroke is more likely to be thrombotic. However, it is difficult to distinguish on clinical grounds, so imaging with CT or MRI is invaluable. Identification of primary cerebral haemorrhage places hypertension firmly at the top of the list of risk factors and also obviates the pursuit of sources of the stroke, as is necessary for a thrombotic event. The thrombotic, or thrombo-embolic, event has more complex and diverse mechanisms: *in situ* pathology in the cerebral arteries, inflammatory vasculitis (either local or proximally), carotid atheroma, aortic disease, cardiac valvular vegetations, atrial and ventricular mural thrombus and paradoxical embolism. These have a wide range of treatment opportunities and warrant additional biochemical and imaging investigation – including carotid ultrasound and Doppler measurement. The distinction between haemorrhagic and thrombotic stroke governs the future use of aspirin as a preventative measure.

Explaining the renal changes

The haematuria, proteinuria and rise in creatinine need explanation. As suggested above, these may relate to renovascular disease – small (and sometimes large) renal infarcts probably account for the haematuria and moderate hypertension for the proteinuria in this circumstance. In the presence of critical renal artery stenoses BP reduction may cause a fall in glomerular filtration – with ACE inhibitors particularly this may progress to renal failure. The question of whether blood detected in the urine arises from the kidneys or a lesion in the bladder can usefully be addressed by microscopic examination of the urine sediment – the presence of tubular casts indicates a glomerular source.

Further interventions

This patient needs his BP well controlled. If the event was thrombotic, low-dose aspirin should be introduced once adequate BP has been achieved. Cholesterol modification with statins is protective against further thrombotic stroke and is also indicated because of his overall vascular risk. He needs strong encouragement to keep off cigarettes. He should diet with the objectives of improving BP control, reducing saturated fat intake, increasing fruit and vegetables, and losing weight.

He should adopt a programme of regular physical activity within the limits of his capabilities – this improves all his other risk factors and in itself reduces recurrent stroke risk.

Case 2

A 43-year-old schoolteacher attends a Monday clinic during the middle of term time. She admits headaches and palpitations. Her BP is 187/122 mmHg and her pulse is 105 beats per minute. The urine dipstix test is normal, there are no vascular changes in the fundi and the ECG shows a sinus tachycardia. Treatment is started straight away with a β-blocker, and she is invited to return later in the week, when her BP is found to be 142/90 mmHg.

She returns to the Monday clinic a few weeks later to collect a further prescription. Symptomatically she feels better, but her BP is again elevated at 190/129 mmHg and her pulse is 98 beats per minute. A 24-hour urinary catecholamine result is available and shows raised excretion values.

- What possible causes of secondary hypertension are suggested, and which of these is most likely?
- What further information do you require to assess her BP?
- How might the differential diagnosis be clarified with relatively simple investigation?
- How would your treatment approach differ from that adopted here?

Discussion

Possible causes of hypertension

This schoolteacher's symptoms and her raised urinary catecholamines indicate that she may have a phaeochromocytoma. The most typical symptom triad includes palpitations, headaches and sweating. Equally, these symptoms may relate to alcohol and particularly the hangover of alcohol withdrawal. Alcohol raises BP and can also cause marked rises in catecholamines, similar to the levels produced by a phaeochromocytoma. Nationally, BP is highest over the weekend and on Mondays, which reflects the habit of binge drinking at weekends, characteristic of the UK and many other populations. It is also worth noting that acute psychoses cause large increases in catecholamines and that treatment with calcium antagonists causes a modest increase. The latter relates to reflex sympathetic activation – and is also associated with headaches and palpitations.

Further information required

A detailed medical history including lifestyle, drugs and medications, is important to assess the hypertensive cause for this patient (recreational drugs – cocaine and amphetamines – also raise catecholamines and are well-recognized causes of acute hypertensive strokes and myocardial ischaemia). However, this woman must be assumed to have a phaeochromocytoma until proven otherwise. But alcohol excess is a far more common and likely explanation.

Investigations

Investigations should include a series of urinary catecholamine measurements, measurement of clues to alcohol excess (γGTP and MCV), blood sugar (because of the diabetogenic effect of catecholamines), calcium and assessment of the thyroid (because of the association of phaeochromocytoma with multiple endocrine adenomas and with medullary carcinoma of the thyroid – family history is particularly important in this context). Definitive investigation requires imaging of the adrenals and the sympathetic chain. An adrenal mass may be identified quickly and simply by ultrasound, if large enough. Optimally, the urgency of this issue warrants an urgent MRI or CT scan.

In this circumstance, initiating treatment with a β-blocker is dangerous as it prevents β-adrenoceptor-mediated vasodilatation and leaves unopposed α-adrenoceptor mediated vasoconstriction. This enhances the severity of a pressor crisis and may prove fatal. In cases in which phaeochromocytoma is suspected, treatment should be initiated with α-blockade – this is most effectively done with phenoxybenzamine in the hands of a specialist – but in general practice doxazosin and urgent referral are appropriate measures. β-blockade can be safely and necessarily introduced to control symptoms and tachycardia after effective α-blockade.

Improving treatment approach

Measuring BP on days other than Monday would help to differentiate the effects of alcohol from phaeocromocytoma. Only if BP is maintained throughout the week would treatment be started, and in view of a suspicion of a phaeocromocytoma, α-blockers rather than β-blocker should be selected.

Case 3

A 59-year-old woman has suffered an inferior myocardial infarction. Acutely, she needed temporary cardiac pacing, but now a month later she is about to return to her job as a restaurateur. Two years ago she suffered a TIA, stopped smoking at the time and has since remained on aspirin 75 mg daily. Now she is 6 kg overweight, her BP is 160/103 mmHg, her pulse 78 beats per minute, and examination of the precordium and chest is normal. She has received no dietary advice.

- What are your treatment objectives here?
- What further information would you like to consider in designing her management?

- What further investigations would you carry out?
- Define the measures you would recommend.

Discussion

Treatment objectives

This woman has suffered both cerebral and coronary artery disease. The treatment objective is that of secondary CVD prevention. This necessitates a comprehensive approach to the relevant risk factors.

Further information and investigations required

It is perhaps a pity that antihypertensive medication was not initiated 2 years ago following the TIA, which should have lowered the threshold for antihypertensive therapy. Treatment with aspirin was appropriate following the TIA, but should have been commenced when the physician was confident of good BP control. Antihypertensive treatment given now might logically include a β-blocker (with concurrent benefit for secondary coronary prevention) and an ACE inhibitor, particularly if there has been any evidence of symptomatic heart failure or ventricular dysfunction on ECG.

Equally, the lipid profile might usefully have been evaluated 2 years ago and the values now need to be obtained. The incidence of myocardial infarction indicates lipid-lowering treatment, but the pattern of total cholesterol, HDL and triglycerides may influence the choice of agents and dosage. To obtain a true reflection of the patient's lipid profile around the time of myocardial infarction the blood sample needs to be taken within 24 hours of the event or otherwise several weeks later. In the postinfarction interval, LDL cholesterol levels, and hence total cholesterol levels, are markedly reduced.

If BP is difficult to control and if renal function is impaired (or creatinine rises following treatment with an ACE inhibitor or angiotensin II antagonist), the possibility of renovascular disease needs to be considered. In an arteriopathic ex-smoker the likelihood of this problem is further enhanced if the patient is diabetic.

Recommended measures

The non-pharmacological measures are very important here – especially in her occupation as a restaurateur. The greatest dietary benefits may be derived from reducing saturated fat intake; beyond this a greener, fresher, more Mediterranean-style diet is advantageous although the particular protective components of this diet remain much debated. She might continue her moderate alcohol intake within the limits of 14 units per week. Weight reduction improves BP – a 2.5/1.5 mmHg fall for each 1 kg weight loss – and also several other risk factors (glucose, cholesterol, fibrinogen, insulin resistance). Weight reduction and regular physical activity are also likely to be strongly protective against further coronary and stroke events.

This woman sensibly gave up smoking following her TIA 2 years ago. She might now be discouraged by the occurrence of the myocardial infarction, in spite of the difficult effort, and consequently be tempted to start smoking again. Anti-smoking advice needs to be strongly reinforced with frequency, even for ex-smokers. In addition to most non-pharmacological measures this woman, like so many others with post-myocardial infarction, will probably need 4 drugs: β-blocker, aspirin, statin and ACE inhibitor.

CASE 4

A patient presents at your surgery with an attack of gout. He is a 56-year-old single accountant who lives alone, and drinks approximately 28 units of alcohol at the weekends. He weighs 78.5 kg, is 1.76 m tall, and his BP is 185/110 mmHg, from three similar recordings on subsequent Monday evening visits to the surgery.

Describe further aspects of history, examination and investigations you require before initiating therapy.

- What measures would you recommend?
- Is drug treatment likely to be necessary?

Discussion

This middle-aged single man is quite likely to have several aspects of his lifestyle that could be usefully corrected. He tends to binge drink at weekends, he is overweight for his height, and has now presented with gout.

Further information and investigations required

The three serial readings of his BP have not shown any tendency to fall with repeated measurements, as is the usual pattern, and may in part at least reflect the weekend alcohol intake. It would be informative to measure his BP later in the week after abstention from alcohol. It will also be very useful to look for evidence of target organ changes. If his BP of 185/100 mmHg was continuously sustained, retinal vascular changes, proteinuria and perhaps ECG changes would be expected. There is an association between gout and hypertension and, of course, treatment of hypertension with thiazide diuretics may precipitate gout. In addition, moderate alcohol consumption and dieting with brisk weight reduction may precipitate gout. A new presentation with gout requires a detailed drug and dietary history, cardiovascular examination, checking for any cause of increased cell turnover such as a lymphoproliferative disorder and a check of thyroid function.

Further information is required about additional risk factors – level of physical activity, family history, cardiovascular history, smoking, blood sugar and cholesterol profile. These aspects influence treatment thresholds and also the choice of antihypertensive agent. If hypertensive target organ change is present, the BP warrants drug treatment straight away without protracted reassessment and regardless of the contributing factors. Transient or episodic hypertension, associated with alcohol or phaeochromocytoma for instance, is less likely to be associated with target organ change.

Unless the patient is a good cook his diet may consist of pre-packaged meals and take-aways – both typically high in salt content. Easily adopted dietary changes may offer enormous benefits. The objectives should be reduction in saturated fat intake, reduction in salt intake, moderation of alcohol and overall reduction in calories. These measures may effectively reduce BP considerably and, in the absence of target organ damage, avoid the need for antihypertensive treatment. In addition, if there are no further acute attacks of gout, specific drug treatment with allopurinol may not be necessary.

Drug therapy

Drug therapy depends on the aetiology of the raised BP on Mondays. If this is induced by alcohol binges and that aspect of lifestyle can be modified, therapy may well not be needed. If these BP levels are maintained throughout the week on repeat measures and the non-pharmacological measures do not lower them to <160/100 mmHg drug therapy is required. As mentioned above, the choice of therapy is influenced by coexisting risk factors and diseases, as are the threshold and targets for starting antihypertensive drugs.

CASE 5

A 62-year-old Caucasian baker, has non-insulin-dependent diabetes. He is taking metformin.

- What are your treatment objectives here?
- What further investigations and information do you require?
- What measures would you adopt?

Case 5 details	
Weight	94 kg
Height	1.72 m
Smokes	15 cigarettes per day
Alcohol intake	56 units per week
BP:	
3 years ago	138/78 mmHg
1 year ago	164/102 mmHg
2 weeks ago	168/104 mmHg
today	168/100 mmHg
Investigations	
Triglycerides	2.7 mmol/l
Total cholesterol	6.3 mmol/l
HDL cholesterol	0.9 mmol/l
Fasting glucose	15 mmol/l (off medication)

Discussion

Treatment objectives

This 62-year-old male, overweight, diabetic smoker with a total:HDL cholesterol ratio of 7.0 carries an enormous cardiovascular risk. The very heavy alcohol intake may protect against coronary disease, but it contributes to the high BP and puts him at increased risk of haemorrhagic stroke. Consequently, the treatment objectives are to prevent a cardiovascular event.

Further investigation required

All routine investigations for hypertension should be carried out (e.g. ECG, electrolytes and creatinine, urine dipstix). It appears that BP has risen since a normal recording taken 3 months previously. Several questions arise:

- Was he 'off the booze' 3 months ago?
- He is overweight with fat arms. Have the more recent BP measurements been taken with an inappropriately small cuff, as opposed to the first measurement being taken with a large cuff?
- Are there signs of hypertensive target organ damage that might corroborate these recent readings and suggest that the first reading was erroneously and, for some reason, spuriously low?
- Were the more recent readings taken by the 'white-coated' doctor and the former reading by the nurse or in his local shopping centre?
- Has he started some new medication, such as nonsteroidal anti-inflammatory drugs (NSAIDs), that may have pushed BP up?
- The rapid development of hypertension might indicate the emergence of a secondary form of hypertension. In the context of a middle-aged male diabetic smoker, renovascular stenosis is a strong possibility. Are there any vascular bruits present?

Measures to adopt

If we accept that he is hypertensive, perhaps because there is retinal vascular change and proteinuria, how do we attempt the challenging task of reducing his overall risk? Clearly, with a high starting level of absolute risk there are major returns to be gained from intervention – perhaps none greater than from persuading him to stop smoking. The other obvious issue is that he needs a comprehensive and ordered approach to all his risk factors. He can take a package of medications on board, but he is unlikely to be able to address the non-pharmacological lifestyle issues all at once. He needs advice on diet, smoking, weight reduction, alcohol and exercise – delivery of this advice in a single session is likely to be off-putting and potentially counterproductive.

Medication includes antihypertensive therapy – assuming the three most recent sets of readings are real – avoiding ACE inhibitors or angiotensin-II receptor antagonists until the suspicion of renovascular disease has been dealt with. The presence of diabetes reduces the threshold for initiating BP treatment to 140/90 mmHg. The target

BP is similarly reduced and yet further reduction to 125/75 mmHg is indicated by the additional complications of proteinuria and retinopathy. Effective antihypertensive therapy to achieve target control is likely to include at least two drugs. The cardinal objective here is tight BP control. Once adequate BP control has been achieved, low-dose aspirin should be introduced. He also needs an aggressive approach to correction of his lipid profile with an adequate dose of a statin, unless the non-drug measures have a large beneficial effect on his lipids (e.g. total:HDL ratio of <4). Lipids and BP are the two most important determinants of adverse outcome in diabetics. The non-pharmacological measures – particularly weight reduction and exercise – also improve these risk factors. He is already taking the appropriate hypoglycaemic agent – metformin – for an overweight type II diabetic. The dosage probably needs to be increased and with time additional agents, including insulin, may be required. Again, the dietary and lifestyle measures are of paramount importance in aiming to improve sugar control.

CASE 6

A 71-year-old widow has been troubled by angina over the past 2 years. She uses glyceryl trinitrate spray + propranolol 40 mg t.d.s. She also has a history of treated hypertension. A month ago your colleague saw her because the patient had noticed swelling of her ankles. He prescribed bendrofluazide 5 mg daily. Now she returns with increasing breathlessness and generally feeling unwell.

- Describe further aspects of the history, examination and investigations you think important.
- What treatment measures would you adopt?

Discussion
Further important information

This elderly woman probably has heart failure. She has two important risk factors for this problem – hypertension and ischaemic heart disease. However, unless the physical signs are obvious (ankle oedema alone is not a very discriminatory feature) the diagnosis is often difficult to make purely on clinical grounds. Echo is extremely helpful in making or refuting the diagnosis, in defining the severity of the problem, and also in evaluating the cause – thickened hypertensive left ventricle, regional wall ischaemia, valvular defect, dilated cardiomyopathy etc.

A further question is 'why has she recently deteriorated?' There are several possibilities:

- BP has been inadequately controlled
- she has had a myocardial infarct
- she has developed atrial fibrillation
- she has started taking medication that enhances sodium and fluid retention, such as NSAIDs or chlorpropamide for diabetes
- she has had a pulmonary embolism; pulmonary embolism causes right ventricular failure and the consequent hypoxia, enhanced sympathetic drive and inadequate coronary perfusion may precipitate left ventricular failure in those with underlying ischaemic disease.

These need further evaluation through examination, Echo and laboratory tests that include a full blood count, cardiac enzymes, thyroid function and renal function, in addition to all the routine tests for a hypertensive patient.

Treatment measures

In any circumstance, good BP control needs to be maintained. The most appropriate agents for the management of hypertension complicated by heart failure are thiazide diuretics, ACE inhibitors and β-blockers.

If left ventricular function is adequate with a reasonable ejection fraction on Echo it may be reasonable to continue the β-blocker (particularly as she has angina), but to switch from propranolol to a longer-acting agent, such as bisoprolol, that has been shown in trials to improve outcome in heart failure patients. When initiating β-blockers for heart failure the maxim is to 'start low and go slow' – that is to titrate up from a low dose over weeks and months. The largest body of evidence supports the use of ACE inhibitors in heart failure – usually in conjunction with a diuretic, as these are particularly effective for acute symptom relief. It is disappointing that only a small proportion of patients with established heart failure are effectively treated with adequate doses of ACE inhibitors. There is also accumulating evidence for the efficacy of AII receptor antagonists in the management of heart failure if ACE inhibitors are not tolerated.

In this woman's case – a common problem of hypertension (often systolic hypertension) complicated by heart failure – thiazide plus ACE inhibitor plus β-blocker may prove an effective combination therapy. In addition, the non-pharmacological measures of weight reduction, regular physical activity and salt restriction make very important contributions to the management of heart failure in the hypertensive patient.

Finally, given that this patient has active ischaemic heart disease, she almost certainly requires lipid-lowering therapy with a statin and, once her BP has been controlled, she will also require low-dose aspirin.

Case 7

A 69-year-old Scotsman develops shortness of breath and is found to be in atrial fibrillation. There are no overt signs of heart failure. The pulse is controlled to 90 beats per minute with digoxin, which produces symptomatic improvement such that he is breathless only on steep hills. His BP measures 155/95 mmHg after three visits, and the fundi show grade 1 hypertensive change.

His past history includes attacks of gout, but he is not on any maintenance therapy. He is athletic – playing tennis and squash until the previous year, and still swims regularly. He is an ex-smoker (40 per day, and stopped at age 35) with a prodigious alcohol intake of 76 units per week. His father died at 76 of prostate cancer; his mother and three maternal aunts died aged 96, 89, 94 and 102 years respectively.

Further data include an ECG that showed atrial fibrillation, no ischaemic changes, no voltage abnormalities, a total cholesterol of 7.7 mmol/l and an HDL of 2.8 mmol/l. His medication is digoxin 0.25 mg once a day and aspirin 150 mg once a day.

- Outline likely causes of his problem.
- What advice needs to be given?
- What treatments should be adopted?

Discussion
Causes of the problem

This man's atrial fibrillation may be driven by hypertension. More than 50% of patients with atrial fibrillation have either current hypertension or a history of hypertension. An inspired guess may lead you to suspect his enormous weekly alcohol intake of 76 units as another contributing factor. The other possible causes that need assessment include risk factors for ischaemic heat disease, thyroid function, valvular heart disease and infection.

His athleticism tends to refute significant ischaemic heart disease, although this supposition may be completely incorrect – many famous athletes have succumbed to sudden myocardial infarctions. He stopped smoking many years ago and the attendant risk for stroke and coronary disease will have largely diminished. There is a remarkable history of longevity on the maternal side of his family and he appears to have inherited the 'survival factor' of an elevated HDL cholesterol, which produces a total:HDL cholesterol ratio of less than 3! Alcohol may also be contributing to his favourable lipid profile.

Advice and treatments required

There is no doubt that he needs to diminish the risk of further gout attacks and reduce his alcohol intake for the sake of his liver as well as his brain!

The risk of thromboembolism related to atrial fibrillation generally warrants anticoagulation with warfarin, even if the interval of atrial fibrillation is only a matter of hours. Warfarin should certainly be instigated before any attempt at cardioversion. However, warfarin anticoagulation in the setting of alcohol excess and an erratic lifestyle may be contraindicated. If BP remains even marginally elevated it should be treated effectively, as this improves the chances of correcting the atrial fibrillation to sinus rhythm.

The greatest benefits here can be achieved by reduction of alcohol intake, control of any residual hypertension, correction of atrial fibrillation (under anticoagulation cover) and continued regular exercise.

CASE 8

A 42-year-old Pakistani accountant is now working in London. She is a non-smoker and drinks no alcohol. She has two older children aged 13 and 9 years and a baby daughter of 4 months. Her recent third pregnancy was complicated by hypertension. She is anxious about her strong family history of CHD and hypertension. A series of BP checks on three occasions shows values of 158–170/92–104 mmHg, and a pulse of 90–108 beats per minute.

- What investigations does she need?
- Predict her body weight and shape and predict her metabolic profile.

- Plan her management; if drugs are required outline your order of preference.

Discussion

Investigations required

This young woman appears to have mild hypertension, and hence all the routine investigations for hypertension are indicated. Anxiety about the consultation and her expressed concerns may well be contributing to the measurements in surgery and additional observations with an ambulatory BP monitor (ABPM) may be helpful. As always, it is important to look for signs of target organ change (examination of the fundi, the heart, ECG, urine dipstix) that may distinguish hypertension from a white-coat response. The occurrence of hypertension in her third pregnancy predicts future essential hypertension, and it may take several weeks and even months to settle to pre-pregnancy levels. This is likely to have been 'late gestational hypertension' rather than pre-eclampsia. The positive family history of hypertension and coronary heart disease also supports the diagnosis.

As hypertension is a common problem, so a family history of hypertension is common, but this finding should not lead to the assumption that the hypertension here is necessarily essential. Particularly in a young patient, possible secondary causes should be considered through examination and appropriate investigation. An important consideration here is the possibility that she may have been started on the combined oral contraceptive (OC) pill. If so, it should be discontinued, if possible, an alternative method of contraception put in place (possibly the progestogen-only pill [POP]), and BP re-assessed.

Body weight, shape and metabolic profile

With her ethnic origin, mild hypertension and family history, this woman is likely to be 'insulin resistant'; as such she may be overweight with central obesity (which may have been enhanced by the recent pregnancy), she may be glucose intolerant and also have a dyslipidaemia characterized by low HDL cholesterol and high triglycerides. Importantly, she is likely to have low or marginal levels of several risk factors and not 'score' in any of the parameters of a standard CVD risk assessment algorithm. Thus her problem may well be underestimated. It is also evident that women and ethnic minorities generally receive inadequate treatment in cardiovascular terms.

Management plan

The principal approach to her management must start with all the non-pharmacological measures – weight reduction, dietary adjustment to reduce saturated fat and salt intake, increased fresh fruit and vegetable intake, and regular physical activity. These proposals may come at a difficult time when she is busy with a young baby.

If hypertension is confirmed with a 24-hour ABPM, medication may be added to the lifestyle measures. It is important to know whether she is breastfeeding and to ensure adequate plans for contraception. Only very small quantities of antihypertensive drugs pass to the baby via breast milk and calcium antagonists (long-acting nifedipine), β-blockers and thiazides are safely used in this circumstance. Given the probable characteristics of insulin resistance here, an α-blocker would be an appropriate choice as a first-line antihypertensive, since this is the only drug group that clearly improves insulin sensitivity. Alternatively, if no further pregnancies are planned and safe contraception is undertaken, an ACE inhibitor could be used.

Case 9

An opportunistic BP check in a 40-year-old housewife shows a level of 195/115 mmHg, and a pulse of 80 beats per minute. She had first used the OC pill at the age of 18 years. She recalls being told that her BP was 'slightly high but nothing to

Laboratory results for Case 9	
Total cholesterol	8.37 mmol/l
HDL cholesterol	1.57 mmol/l
Triglycerides	1.69 mmol/l
Fasting glucose	Normal
Creatinine	116 (μmol/l
Sodium	138 mmol/l
Potassium	3.7 mmol/l

worry about'. She has two children aged 20 and 15 years, and no comment was made about her BP in either pregnancy. She used the OC for two prolonged spells. A few years ago she restarted the OC (ethinyloestradiol with gestodene). Regular BP checks showed that it was frequently mildly elevated. She said that she had always been terrified of having her BP measured. She has a history of migraine since her teens, and smokes 20 cigarettes per day. She does not drink alcohol and takes no exercise. She is frequently 'on a diet'. Her mother (aged 63 years) is hypertensive, is on medication and has had coronary bypass surgery and bilateral carotid endarterectomy.

Examination shows that the patient is overweight by about 15 kg (body mass index, 31.3). There are no indications of hypertensive target organ change – in particular the urine dipstix is normal and the fundi look normal. The ECG is normal. Laboratory results are given above.

- Describe your plan for her management.

Discussion

The management plan for this woman could be considered under three headings:

- immediate interventions – non-pharmacological advice
- further investigations
- what drugs (if any) are required, and when.

Immediate interventions

Despite being a premenopausal woman she is at significant risk of a cardiovascular event by virtue of several risk factors in combination:

- heavy smoker
- high BP
- adverse lipid profile – the total cholesterol:HDL ratio isn't too bad (5.3), but the total cholesterol is too high and her calculated LDL cholesterol is raised
- migraine – this condition more than trebles the risk of ischaemic stroke
- OC use – in a woman of this type, the risk of a major CV event is more than doubled by her oral contraceptive
- positive family history of cardiovascular disease – on average this increases her risk by about 50%
- overweight, no exercise and no alcohol, all of which are associated with increased cardiovascular risk.

Taking all these considerations into account, her relative cardiovascular risk is at least 50 times higher than that of her peers. Consequently, her absolute risk is a real consideration.

As her migraine and family history are not modifiable, effort should be directed at improving her modifiable risk factors – quickly!

Rapid risk reduction would be achieved by stopping smoking and, at the end of her current cycle, her OC. Hence advice and counselling on both of these risk factors must be supplied. If the patient is desperate to stay on an OC, this could be negotiated once her smoking habit, body weight, lipid levels and exercise level have improved. At this point the combined OC should be replaced by a POP.

The next priorities after smoking and OC use are to reduce her weight and change her lipid profile. Both will be greatly improved by reducing total and saturated fat intakes, and appropriate advice should be supplied. Gradually increasing aerobic exercise enhances the benefits of weight loss and fat restriction. The patient should also be encouraged to replace her fatty foods with fresh fruit and vegetables.

Investigations

The combination of high BP readings, normal fundi and urine and the admission of 'terror' when having BP measured raises the possibility of some degree of white-coat hypertension. Hence investigations should be set up to evaluate that possibility. In addition, in view of the severe BP levels recorded, other tests to exclude secondary causes of hypertension should be arranged. Hence she requires:

- several repeat clinic BPs
- 24-hour ABPM
- Echo (chronic, genuine BPs of 195/118 mmHg will produce some degree of LVH)
- 24-hour urinary catecholamines to exclude phaeochromocytoma
- plasma aldosterone and renin to consider alongside her electrolytes for an evaluation of possible Conn's syndrome
- some investigation for renal artery stenosis; renal angiogram is definitive, but invasive and expensive, so a renal ultrasound and plasma renin measurement may be a reasonable starting point.

Drug therapy

The question arises whether to defer treatment of her BP levels until the ABPM and Echo have been carried out. Given her age and high relative and absolute risk, it is probably wise to repeat clinic BP measurements over 1–2 weeks and, if they are still raised, start treatment pending ABPM and Echo results. Several considerations influence the choice of drugs – young women often do not like the urinary problems that may be associated with diuretics and her dyslipidaemia also mitigates against their use. β-blockers may be useful insofar as they may improve her migraines and anxiety (if white-coat hypertension is demonstrated it may reflect a general tendency). As ACE inhibitors should perhaps be deferred until renal artery stenosis has been excluded, either a dihydropyridine calcium antagonist or an α-blocker may be suitable.

It may be prudent to recommend aspirin use during any or all migraine attacks, but not otherwise since young hypertensive women are more prone to haemorrhagic than ischaemic strokes.

Regarding her contraception, as mentioned above, until her risk levels are greatly reduced she should ideally stop her combined OC. Re-starting oral contraception could be considered, but a POP should be used.

Finally, the possibility of lipid-lowering therapy should be considered. Using, for example, the New Zealand risk chart, this woman is at about 5% risk of a cardiovascular event in the next 5 years. However, this risk score does not incorporate her family history, migraine and lack of exercise. These considerations certainly raise her absolute risk to 15% over the next 5 years.

However, with appropriate dietary and other lifestyle manoeuvres along with BP reduction, this risk can be significantly reduced and, assuming such manoeuvres are effective, the use of a statin could reasonably be deferred.

Case 10

A 52-year-old woman attends complaining of hot flushes and vaginal dryness. Her BP is 175/105 mmHg, her fundi are grade 2 with A-V nipping, she smokes 10 cigarettes per day, drinks 2 units of alcohol per week and she is thin. Her father died of myocardial infarct at 54 years of age, and her mother died at 96 years of age. Her ECG is 'normal', as are her creatinine and electrolytes, and her total cholesterol is 7.7 mmol/l.

- What advice and treatments may be considered?

Discussion

The advice and treatments for this woman can be considered under two headings:

- those relating to her presenting complaint
- those relating to her cardiovascular risk.

Presenting complaint

Hot flushes, which may be variably debilitating, remain a key indication for prescribing HRT. If she has had a hysterectomy the HRT should be 'unopposed' (oestrogen only). If not it should be a combined (oestrogen and progestogen) formulation. On average, HRT does not raise BP, although in a very small proportion of women marked hypertension following the use of HRT has been reported. Hence BP should always be monitored following the initiation of HRT.

In the postmenopausal woman the role of HRT for CVD prevention had been advocated on the basis of several observational reports. These may well have been unrepresentative because the most enthusiastic users of HRT were women from social classes I and II – the 'worried well' – with a relatively healthy lifestyle and hence low levels of coronary risk. The results of the HERS trial, which allocated women with high levels of CVD risk (post myocardial infarction) to either placebo or oestrogen replacement therapy, show that HRT has no benefit in terms of CVD prevention. The trial was prospective, randomized and blinded. The indications for use of HRT in postmenopausal women therefore remain those of controlling symptoms related to oestrogen deficiency and reducing the risk of osteoporosis. The pragmatic approach to HRT among women who have started it in anticipation of cardiovascular benefit may be to continue if they are comfortable, if they are aware of the risks and if there are no specific contraindications. The results of the HERS trial, while being an important negative, should not engender panic.

Cardiovascular risk

In addition to the cardiovascular implications of HRT use discussed above, this women has several cardiovascular risk factors:

- hypertension (the A-V nipping confirms this diagnosis)
- smoker
- family history of myocardial infarction
- elevated total cholesterol.

Using the New Zealand risk chart to calculate her risk (assuming she is not diabetic, and has an HDL cholesterol of 1.1 mmol/l) she has a 5-year risk of a cardiovascular event of between 10–15%, but allowing for her family history this increases to about 15–25%. This is clearly unacceptable and requires intervention. However, the patient requires further evaluation.

Other requirements

All hypertensive patients should also have, as part of a minimal investigation, a urine dipstix test for protein and blood, a glucose measurement and a lipid evaluation, which should also include HDL cholesterol (this can be carried out without fasting). A full blood count (for MCV) and a γGTP are also often carried out to help to confirm or refute the alcohol history. From the results of these tests, a more accurate cardiovascular risk estimate can be made.

Meanwhile, non-pharmacological advice should be supplied to lower her cardiovascular risk and a series of paired BP readings could be taken to confirm her hypertensive status. The advice should include:

- stop smoking
- reduce salt intake

- decrease total and saturated fat intake
- increase fresh fruit and vegetable intake.

Given her A-V nipping it is unlikely that her BP will be adequately controlled (i.e. to <140/85 mmHg) by nondrug measures unless she turned out to be an alcoholic who stopped drinking. Consequently, antihypertensive medication needs to be selected. Her probable dyslipidaemia makes diuretics or β-blockers possibly less suitable than metabolically friendly drugs, such as an ACE inhibitor, a CCB, or an α-blocker.

However, any of these five drug groups could be used, and it is quite likely she will need at least two drugs to provide good BP control.

The HRT is likely to produce some improvement in her lipid profiles, but the possibility of lipid lowering should also be considered. If this woman can be persuaded to stop smoking and adopt moderate dietary changes and (say to produce a total HDL cholesterol ratio of 6), assuming her BP is reduced to 140/85 mmHg, then her 5-year CV risk falls to about 6%. If this is achieved, lipid-lowering drugs would not be indicated. However if, despite her best efforts, she remained with a 5-year CV risk of >15%, many physicians would also add a statin to her therapy.

chapter 12

Trials: past, present and future

The field of hypertension has more large randomized controlled trials to evaluate the impact of interventions on morbidity and mortality than almost any other area of medicine.

Until the mid-1990s all of the major trials to evaluate the effects of BP lowering on morbidity and mortality used either diuretics or β-blockers as first-line agents. The combined results of most of these trials, which included about 47 000 hypertensive patients, have been meta-analysed (Fig. 12.1) [1]. This analysis revealed that a reduction of 5–6 mmHg in diastolic BP was associated with about a 38% reduction in stroke risk and about a 16% reduction in CHD risk. While the effect on stroke reduction was in keeping with prospective observational data, the effect on CHD was rather less than the epidemiological data predicted (Fig. 12.2) [2].

Despite this extensive body of evidence there remained many aspects of the management of hypertension that could not be guided by evidence from randomized controlled trials.

The major omission among the data available by the mid-1990s was evidence regarding the effects on morbidity and mortality of the 'newer' classes of BP-lowering agents (calcium antagonists, ACE inhibitors, α-blockers and angiotensin II antagonists). Since then, however, the SYST-Eur [3], CAPPP [4], UKPDS [5] and other trials have contributed evidence of varying quality to this area. SYST-EUR [3] was the first trial to demonstrate clear benefits on morbidity and mortality associated with

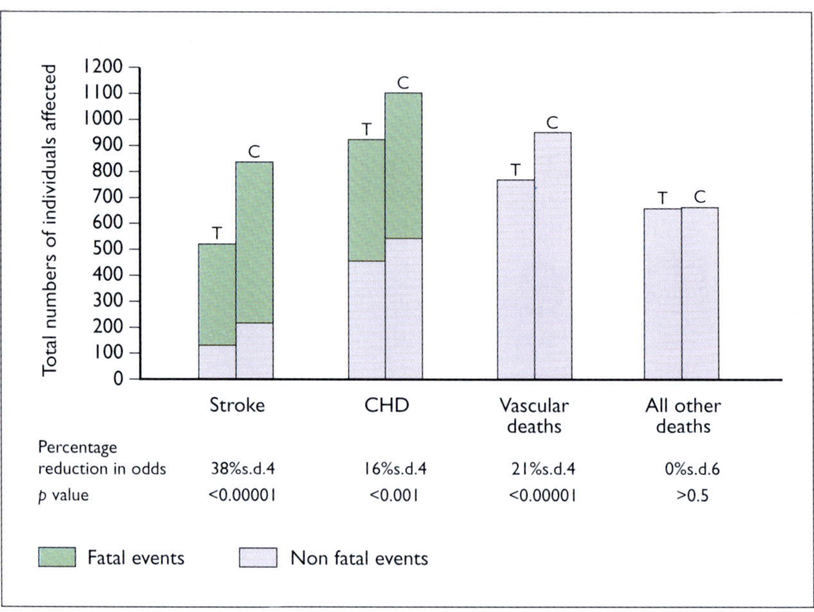

Figure 12.1. Effects of BP reduction on stroke, CHD, vascular death and nonvascular death. Combined results of 17 randomized trials of antihypertensive treatment. T, treatment; C, control.

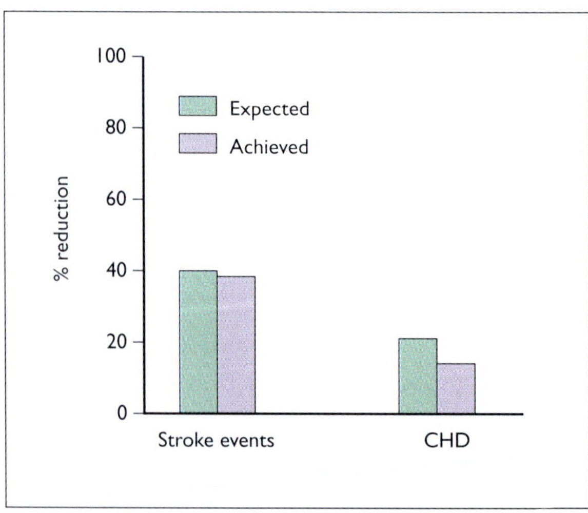

Figure 12.2. Expected versus achieved effects of BP lowering on reduction of stroke and CHD events.

the use of drugs other than diuretics and β-blockers. This trial compared a dihydropyridine calcium antagonist (nitrendipine) versus placebo in older men and women with isolated systolic hypertension.

A further shortcoming of most of the earlier trials was the type of patient included. In general, patients with other major risk factors and comorbidity were excluded. Consequently, optimal therapy for most subgroups of patients, such as those with diabetes, LVH, renal impairment or post-stroke, remained unevaluated.

Some of the more recently published trials have not enforced such rigorous exclusion criteria and hence subgroup analyses have allowed some evaluation of the effects of various drugs in specific subgroups (e.g. diabetes in SYST-EUR [3], CAPPP [4] and Hypertension Optimal Treatment [HOT] [6]). These studies tend to contradict earlier, rather less robust data and showed ACE inhibitors and calcium antagonists are effective agents for diabetic patients with hypertension.

Evidence from the HOT and UKPDS trials have reinforced prospective epidemiological data that targets for BP reduction should be reduced – at least in subgroups such as diabetic patients and those with CHD. The implication of these data is that most patients are likely to need at least two drugs to reach the new, lower targets recommended by all the most recent guidelines for hypertension management.

The HOT study shed light on the benefits of aspirin along with antihypertensive management. In short, while low-dose aspirin reduced total cardiovascular events by 15% – a saving of 53 events –59 extra major bleeds were associated with the use of aspirin. Hence, in primary prevention aspirin should probably only be used for higher risk older patients (>50 years) with controlled hypertension.

In addition to these recently published trials a registry of major ongoing or planned randomized trials – each of which includes at least 1000 patients in each randomized group – has been established [7] and now includes over 30 trials of which the vast majority are yet to publish results. These trials are summarized in Table 12.1. This huge collaboration will allow meta-analysed evaluations of different agents in specific subgroups of patients for whom individual trial evidence is inadequate.

Table 12.1. Characteristics of trials identified as eligible included in the WHO-ISH Trialist collaboration [7]*

	Acronym	Patients (n)	Planned follow-up (years)	Randomized treatments (factorial assignments)	Completion date
1	AASK	1200	5	ACE, β-blocker, DCA (more, less)	2001
2	ABCD	950	5	ACE, DCA	1998
3	ALLHAT	40,000	6	ACE, α-blocker (discontinued), DCA, diuretic (CHOL, open)	2002
4	ANBP2	6000	5	ACE, diuretic	2002
5	ASCOT	18,000	5	DCA with/without ACE, β-blocker with/without diuretic (CHOL, placebo)	2003
6	BENEDICT	2400	3	ACE, NCA, placebo	2001
7	CAPPP	10,800	5	ACE, β-blocker/diuretic	1998
8	CONVINCE	15,000	5	NCA, β-blocker/diuretic	2001
9	CSGTEI	1650	3	AIIA, DCA, placebo	2000
10	DIAB-HYCAR	4000	3	ACE, placebo	1999
11	ELSA	2251	4	DCA, β-blocker	2000
12	HDS	1148	8.2	ACE, β-blocker, open (insulin, sulphonamide, diet)	1998
13	HOPE	9541	4.7	ACE, placebo (vitamin E, placebo)	2000
14	HOT	19,196	3.5	More, less (aspirin, placebo)	1997
15	HYVET	2100	5	ACE, diuretic, placebo	2001
16	INSIGHT	6592	3	DCA, diuretic	1999
17	LIFE	9194	4	AIIA, β-blocker	2001
18	NICS-EH	1000	5	DCA, diuretic	1997
19	NORDIL	11,000	5	NCA, β-blocker/diuretic	2002
20	PART2	617	4	ACE, placebo	1998
21	PHYLLIS	450	3	ACE, placebo (CHOL, placebo)	2000
22	PREVENT	825	5	DCA, placebo	1997
23	PROGRESS	6000	5	ACE, placebo	2000
24	QUIET	1750	3	ACE, placebo	1996
25	RENAAL	1500	4	AIIA, placebo	2002
26	SCOPE	4000	2.5	AIIA, placebo	2003
27	SHELL	4800	3.5	DCA, diuretic	1999
28	STOP-2	6628	4	ACE, β-blocker / diuretic, DCA	1998
29	SYST-EUR	4695	1.6	DCA, placebo	1997
30	VHAS	1414	2	NCA, diuretic	1996

* see acronym key to follow on pp. 256. ACE, angiotensin converting enzyme inhibitor; AIIA, angiotensin II antagonist; ACHD, angiographic coronary heart disease; CHOL, cholesterol lowering; CIT, carotid intimal thickness; CVD, cardiovascular disease; DCA, dihydropyridine calcium antago-

	Patient characteristics				Projected events	
	Entry criteria	Age (years)	Diastolic BP (mmHg)	Systolic BP (mmHg)	Coronary heart disease	Stroke
1	HBP plus renal disease	18–70	≥95	Any	144	72
2	Diabetes	40–74	Any	No ISH	119	59
3	HPB plus CVD risk	>55	90–109	140–179	2580	2790
4	HBP	65–84	≥90	≥160	300	150
5	HBP plus CVD risk	40–79	≥90	≥140	1150	400
6	Diabetes	≥40	≥90	≥140	200	100
7	HBP	25-66	≥100	Any	324	162
8	HBP plus CVD risk	≥55	90–109	140–189	1250	750
9	Diabetes plus proteinuria	30–70	≥85	≥135	124	62
10	Diabetes plus proteinuria	> 50	Any	Any	300	150
11	HBP	45–75	95–115	150–209	89	44
12	HBP plus diabetes	25–75	≥85	≥150	244	122
13	CVD risk	≥55	Any	Any	1200	550
14	HBP	50–80	100–115	Any	552	276
15	HBP	> 80	90–109	160–219	683	341
16	HBP plus CVD risk	55–80	≥95	≥150	246	123
17	HBP plus LVH	55–80	95–115	160–200	693	347
18	HBP	≥60	<115	160–219	30	15
19	HBP	50–69	≥100	Any	360	180
20	Atherosclerosis	18–75	Any	Any	40	14
21	CIT	45–70	95–115	151–210	7	4
22	ACHD	30–80	Any	Any	20	6
23	Stroke or TIA	Any	Any	Any	600	300
24	ACHD	18–75	Any	Any	500	350
25	Diabetes	31–70	<110	<200	100	50
26	HBP	70–89	90–99	160–179	60	30
27	HBP	≥60	<95	161–219	101	50
28	HBP	70–84	≥105	≥180	318	167
29	ISH	≥60	<95	160–219	500	250
30	HBP	40–65	≥95	≥160	40	20

nist; HBP, high blood pressure; ISH, isolated systolic hypertension; less, less intensive blood pressure lowering; LVH, left ventricular hypertrophy; more, more intensive blood pressure lowering; NCA, nondihydropyridine calcium antagonist; open, open control; TIA, transient ischaemic attack.

Key to Table 12.1

1 African American Study of Kidney Disease and Hypertension
2 Appropriate Blood Pressure Control in Diabetes Trial
3 Antihypertensive Therapy and Lipid Lowering Heart Attack Prevention Trial
4 Australian National Blood Pressure Study 2
5 Anglo-Scandinavian Cardiac Outcomes Trial
6 Bergamo Nephrology Diabetes Complication Trial
7 Captopril Prevention Project
8 Controlled Onset Verapamil Investigation for Cardiovascular Endpoints
9 Collaborative Study Group Trial on Effect of Irbesartan
10 Diabetes Hypertension Cardiovascular Morbidity–Mortality and Ramipril
11 European Lacidipine Study of Atherosclerosis
12 Hypertension in Diabetes Study
13 Heart Outcomes Prevention Evaluation Study
14 Hypertension Optimal Treatment Trial
15 Hypertension in the Very Elderly Trial
16 International Nifedipine Gastrointestinal Therapeutic System Study Intervention as a Goal for Hypertension Therapy
17 Losartan Intervention for Endpoint Reduction in Hypertension
18 National Intervention Cooperative Study in Elderly Hypertensives
19 Nordic Diltiazem Study
20 Prevention of Atherosclerosis with Ramipril
21 Plaque Hypertension Lipid Lowering Italian Study
22 Prospective Randomized Evaluation of Vascular Effects of Norvasc
23 Perindopril Protection Against Recurrent Stroke Study
24 Quinapril Ischaemia Event Trial
25 Randomized Evaluation of Noninsulin-dependent Diabetes Mellitus with the Angiotensin II Antagonist Losartan
26 Study of Cognition and Prognosis in Elderly Patients with Hypertension
27 Systolic Hypertension in the Elderly Lacidipine Long-term Study
28 Swedish Trial in Old Patients with Hypertension
29 Systolic Hypertension in Europe Multicentre Trial
30 Verapamil in Hypertension Atherosclerosis Study

Clearly, with the publication of the results of these trials, our knowledge of the benefits of certain drug groups among specific subgroups of patients (e.g. those with LVH from the Losartan Intervention for Endpoint Reduction [LIFE] [8] and the very elderly from the Hypertension in the Very Elderly Trial [HYVET] [9]) will be greatly enhanced. Furthermore, studies such as the Antihypertensive and Lipid Lowering Treatment to Prevent Heart Attack Trial (ALLHAT) [10] and Anglo-Scandinavian Cardiac Outcomes Trial (ASCOT) [11] will provide more definitive evidence regarding the benefits or otherwise of the newer agents compared with the standard first-line agents (β-blockers or diuretics), particularly with respect to CHD. However, to date the ASCOT study [11] is the only trial designed to compare the effects of the standard β-blocker plus diuretic combination with a more contemporary regimen (dihydropyridine calcium antagonist plus ACE inhibitor). Further trials to evaluate and compare the effects of different drug combinations are clearly needed, given the current recommendations for more aggressive BP lowering, which will inevitably result in the increased use of two or more drugs.

As cardiovascular disease prevention moves towards a more holistic management approach, several hypertension trials have been designed to evaluate the benefits of additional interventions along with various antihypertensive regimens (ASCOT and ALLHAT [statins], International Nifedipine Gastrointestinal Therapeutic System Study Intervention as a Goal in Hypertension Treatment [INSIGHT] [12] and Heart Outcome Prevention Evaluation [HOPE] [13] [antioxidants])

With publication of the results of all the ongoing trials and the added benefit of the prospective collaborative overview of the major randomized trials of BP-lowering treatments [7], the first decade of the twenty-first century will be an even more exciting time for CVD prevention than the 1990s.

REFERENCES

1. Collins R, Peto R, MacMahon S, *et al.* Blood pressure, stroke, and coronary heart disease. Part 2, short-term reductions in blood pressure: overview of randomised drug trials in their epidemiological context. *Lancet* 1990; **335**: 827–39.
2. MacMahon S, Peto R, Cutler J, *et al.* Blood pressure, stroke, and coronary heart disease. Part I, prolonged differences in blood pressure: prospective observational studies corrected for the regression dilution bias. *Lancet* 1990; **335**: 765–74.
3. Staessen JA, Fagard R, Thijs L, *et al.*, for the Systolic Hypertension-Europe (Syst-Eur) Trial Investigators. Morbidity and mortality in the placebo-controlled European Trial on Isolated Systolic Hypertension in the Elderly. *Lancet* 1997; **350**: 757–64.
4. Hansson L, Lindholm LH, Niskanen L, *et al.* Effect of angiotensin-converting enzyme inhibition compared with conventional therapy on cardiovascular morbidity and mortality in hypertension: the Captopril Prevention Project (CAPPP). *Lancet* 1999; **353**: 611–15.
5. United Kingdom Prospective Diabetes Study Group. Tight blood pressure control and risk of macrovascular and microvascular complications in type 2 diabetes. UKPDS 38. *Br Med J* 1998; **317**; 703–13.
6. Hansson L, Zanchetti A, Carruthers SG, *et al.* for the HOT Study Group. Effects of intensive blood-pressure lowering and low-dose aspirin in patients with hypertension: principal results of the Hypertension Optimal Treatment (HOT) randomised trial. *Lancet* 1998; **351**: 1755–62.
7. World Health Organization–International Society of Hypertension Blood Pressure Lowering Treatment Trialists' Collaboration. Protocol for prospective collaborative overviews of major randomized trials of blood-pressure-lowering treatments. *J Hypertens* 1998; **16**: 127–37.
8. Dahlof B, Devereux R, de Faire U, *et al.* for the LIFE Study Group. The Losartan Intervention for Endpoint Reduction (LIFE) in Hypertension Study. Rationale, design, and methods. *J Hypertens* 1997; **10**: 705–13.
9. Bulpitt C, Fletcher A, Amery A, *et al.* The hypertension in the very elderly trial (HYVET). *Drugs Ageing* 1994; **5**: 171–83.
10. Davis BR, Cutler JA, Gordon DJ, *et al.* Rationale and design for the antihypertensive and lipid lowering treatment to prevent heart attack trial (ALLHAT). *Am J Hypertens* 1996; **9**: 342–60.

11. Dahlof B, Sever PS, Poulter NR, Wedel H. On behalf of the ASCOT Steering Committee. International Society of Hypertension. *J Hypertens* 1998; **16** (Suppl. 2): S212.
12. Brown MJ, Castaigne A, de-Leeuw PW, *et al.* Influence of diabetes and type of hypertension on response to antihypertensive treatment. *Hypertension* 2000; **35(5)**: 1038–42.
13. Heart Outcome Prevention Evaluation (HOPE) Study Investigators. Effects of ramipril on cardiovascular on cardiovascular and microvascular outcomes in people with diabetes mellitus: results of the HOPE study and MICRO-HOPE substudy. *Lancet* 2000; **355**: 253–59.

Index

A

B

T

U

V

W